AAOS
AMERICAN ACADEMY OF ORTHOPAEDIC SURGEONS

ECSI

EMERGENCY CARE
& SAFETY INSTITUTE

Wilderness
FIRST AID
FIELD GUIDE SECO

Alton L. Thygerson
EdD, FAWM

Steven M. Thygerson
PhD, MSPH

Benjamin Gulli
MD, FAAOS
Medical Editor

JONES & BARTLETT
LEARNING

World Headquarters
Jones & Bartlett Learning
5 Wall Street
Burlington, MA 01803
978-443-5000
info@jblearning.com
www.jblearning.com

Jones & Bartlett Learning books and products are available through most bookstores and online booksellers. To contact Jones & Bartlett Learning directly, call 800-832-0034, fax 978-443-8000, or visit our website, www.jblearning.com.

Substantial discounts on bulk quantities of Jones & Bartlett Learning publications are available to corporations, professional associations, and other qualified organizations. For details and specific discount information, contact the special sales department at Jones & Bartlett Learning via the above contact information or send an email to specialsales@jblearning.com.

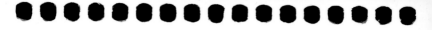

Production Credits
Chief Executive Officer: Ty Field
President: James Homer
Chief Product Officer: Eduardo Moura
VP, Executive Publisher: Kimberly Brophy
Executive Editor: Christine Emerton
Editorial Specialist: Jennifer Meltz
Production Editor: Cindie Bryan
VP, Sales—Public Safety Group: Matthew Maniscalco
Director of Sales, Public Safety Group: Patricia Einstein
VP, Marketing: Alisha Weisman
VP, Manufacturing and Inventory Control: Therese Connell
Art Development Editor: Joanna Lundeen
Composition: Cenveo Publisher Services
Cover and Text Design: Kristin E. Parker
Manager of Photo Research, Rights & Permissions: Lauren Miller
Cover Image: © Peter Kunasz/ShutterStock, Inc.
Printing and Binding: John P. Pow Company

and has not been authorized, sponsored, or otherwise approved by the owners of the trademarks or service marks referenced in this product.

The procedures and protocols in this book are based on the most current recommendations of responsible medical sources. The American Academy of Orthopaedic Surgeons and the publisher, however, make no guarantee as to, and assume no responsibility for, the correctness, sufficiency, or completeness of such information or recommendations. Other or additional safety measures may be required under particular circumstances.

This textbook is intended solely as a guide to the appropriate procedures to be employed when rendering emergency care to the sick and injured. It is not intended as a statement of the standards of care required in any particular situation, because circumstances and the patient's physical condition can vary widely from one emergency to another. Nor is it intended that this textbook shall in any way advise emergency personnel concerning legal authority to perform the activities or procedures discussed. Such local determination should be made only with the aid of legal counsel.

ISBN: 978-1-284-21265-5

Library of Congress Cataloging-in-Publication Data

Thygerson, Alton L.
  Wilderness first aid field guide / Alton L. Thygerson, Steven M. Thygerson, Matthew L. Thygerson, American Academy of Orthopaedic Surgeons, Wilderness Medical Society, Boy Scouts of America. — Second edition.
      pages cm
  Includes bibliographical references.
  ISBN 978-1-4496-4221-1 (pbk.) — ISBN 1-4496-4221-7 (pbk.)
1. Mountaineering injuries.   2. Outdoor medical emergencies.   3. First aid in illness and injury.   I. Title.
  RC88.9.M6 T49 2014
  617.1'0276522—dc23
                                                                    2014040295

6048
Printed in the United States of America
20 19 18 17 16   10 9 8 7 6 5 4

Contents

Leaves: © javarman/ShutterStock, Inc.

A–Z of Injuries and Sudden Illnesses   33

F   107

H   114

■ S   145

■ T   155

■ W   158

■ Prevention   159

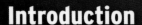

Introduction

Leaves: © javarman/ShutterStock, Inc.

Everyone should be prepared for injuries and medical problems when in situations (e.g., the wilderness) in which professional medical care is not readily available. The Wilderness Medical Society defines "wilderness" as being more than 1 hour away from definitive medical care. Thus, you may be in a wilderness environment without realizing it. Some activities, places, and events that can cause you to be in a wilderness situation include the following:

- Personal recreation (e.g., campers, hikers, hunters, rafters, birders, skiers, and climbers)
- Remote occupations (e.g., farmers, foresters, linesmen, and ranchers)
- Remote residences (e.g., small communities, farms, ranches, and vacation homes)
- Remote locations (e.g., remote parts of North America and developing countries)
- Disasters (e.g., winter storms, hurricanes, earthquakes, tornadoes, and floods)

Those far from medical help may be confronted with the following:

- Delayed or prolonged evacuation because of bad weather, a difficult location, or a lack of transportation or communication
- Adverse conditions (e.g., heat, cold, rain, snow, and altitude)
- Limited first aid supplies and equipment (e.g., restricted to portable and/or improvisation)
- Injuries and illnesses not typically seen in urban areas (e.g., altitude illness, frostbite, and wild animal attacks)
- The need for advanced care (e.g., reducing some dislocations and wound care)
- The need to make difficult decisions (e.g., CPR and evacuation)

The purpose of this guide is to prepare you for victim assessment and care in all of these situations. It contains current emergency care recommendations from the Wilderness Medical Society's *Practice Guidelines for Wilderness Emergency Care,* the Wilderness Medical Society and American Academy of Orthopaedic Surgeons' book *Wilderness First Aid: Emergency Care in Remote Locations,* protocols from the National Association of EMS Physicians and the State of Alaska Cold Injuries Guidelines, and current medical literature.

These guidelines should not be considered final, as they will be constantly updated to reflect current standards of care. The authors and publisher will not be held responsible, nor

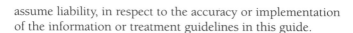

assume liability, in respect to the accuracy or implementation of the information or treatment guidelines in this guide.

Abbreviations/Mnemonics Used

AVPU = alert and aware, responds to voice, responds to pain, unresponsive

CPR = cardiopulmonary resuscitation

DOTS = deformity, open wounds, tenderness, swelling

SAMPLE = symptoms, which are the physical and mental features of an illness or injury as described by the victim, including the chief complaint; allergies; medications; pertinent past history; last oral intake; and events leading up to the illness or injury

RICE = rest, ice, compression, elevation

ASAP = as soon as possible

Signaling for Help

Many emergency conditions require a search for people in distress. Under such circumstances, it is always better if those being sought know how to make their presence and location conspicuous.

Signaling Aircraft

The key to any ground signal is that very few straight lines or right angles exist in nature. Remember that things appear a lot smaller when viewed from the air, and thus, bigger is almost always better. For ground signals, make a large **V** for immediate assistance or an **X** if medical assistance is needed. Make the lines of these signals as large as you can.

Construct your signal using a ratio of six to one (e.g., a **V** with sides 12 × 2 feet). Contrast is another key to ground signals. Examples of materials to use include toilet paper, strips of plastic tarp, strips of tent material, tree branches, logs, and light-colored rocks. In snow, on the open ground, or on a beach, signals may be tramped or dug into the surface using shadows to make the signals stand out.

Other Signals

A series of three signals in quick succession indicates "help." Examples include three shouts, three shots, three blasts from a whistle, and three flashes from a light.

Use smoke by day and bright flame by night if other signaling devices are not available. Add engine oil, rags soaked in oil, or pieces of rubber to your fire to make black smoke (best against light background). Add green leaves, moss, or a little water to send up billows of white smoke (best against dark background). If tending a fire while waiting for help, keep plenty of fuel at hand. Throw it on the fire the moment an aircraft is heard—it takes time for smoke to form and rise.

A mirror is an effective means of sending a distress signal. On hazy days, an aircraft can see the flash of a mirror before survivors can see the aircraft; it is wise to flash the mirror in the direction of a plane when you hear it, even if you cannot see it. Mirror flashes have been spotted by rescue aircraft more than 20 miles away.

To use a mirror, follow this procedure:

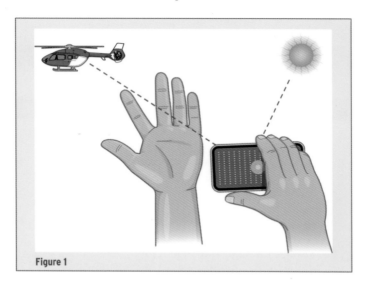

Figure 1

1. Hold the mirror up to the sun with one hand, and stretch your other hand in front of you, holding up a finger or thumb so that it blots out the view of your target.
2. Hit your extended finger or thumb with a reflection of the sun from the mirror.
3. Repeatedly flick the spot of light from the mirror across the finger or thumb and the aircraft.
4. Try to hit the aircraft or rescuers with a flash as much as possible. **DO NOT** attempt to do a series of three flashes—it is too difficult. **Figure 1**

■ Evacuation*

A victim's health or survival may depend on moving him/her to medical care. Determining the best method (e.g., helicopter versus carrying versus walking) must be based on several factors:

- Severity of the illness or injury
- Rescue skill and medical skill of rescuers
- Physical and psychological condition of rescuers and victim
- Availability of equipment and aid for the rescue
- Amount of time—determined by distance, terrain, weather, and other conditions—that it would take to evacuate the victim
- Cost

* This is adapted from and based on the Wilderness Medical Society's *Practice Guidelines for Wilderness Emergency Care.*

It is usually best to postpone further travel and/or initiate evacuation from the wilderness for any person who has the following:

- Worsening symptoms, such as:
  - Altered mental status
  - Unrelieved vomiting or diarrhea
  - An inability to tolerate drinking fluids
  - Losing consciousness for a second time after a head injury

- Debilitating pain
- Inability to travel at a reasonable pace because of a medical problem
- Sustained abdominal pain
- Passage of blood by mouth or rectum (not from an obviously minor source)
- Serious high-altitude illness signs and symptoms
- Infections that worsen despite appropriate treatment
- Chest pain that is not clearly musculoskeletal in origin
- Development of a dysfunctional psychological status that impairs the safety of the person or group
- Large or severe wounds or a wound with complications (e.g., open fracture, deformed fracture, a suspected spinal injury, a fracture or dislocation impairing circulation to arm or leg)

Guidelines for Helicopter Evacuation

Helicopters can reduce the time to medical care. Evacuate by helicopter only if the following applies:

- The victim's life will be saved.
- The victim will have a significantly better chance for full recovery.
- The pilot believes conditions are safe enough for helicopter evacuation.
- Ground evacuation would be dangerous or prolonged, or lacks a sufficient number of rescuers.

Helicopter Safety Rules

The main hazards are the main rotor blades and the tail rotor (appears nearly invisible during operation).

- Always approach the helicopter from the front where the pilot can see you.
- Never walk downhill to approach the helicopter. Never walk uphill when exiting a helicopter.
- Board only when the pilot approves.
- Secure all loose clothing and equipment.
- Never chase an item that has blown away. Wait for the helicopter to land.

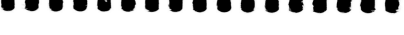

- Protect eyes from the rotor downwash. If blinded by debris, stop and kneel. Someone will come to help.
- **DO NOT** stand in the landing zone.
- Clear debris from the landing zone before the helicopter's arrival.

Guidelines for Ground Evacuation

If the victim is walking out, at least two people should accompany him or her. If the victim is unable to continue, one person can stay with the victim while the other goes for help.

If the victim is being carried out:

- Send someone to notify authorities that help is needed.
- At least four, preferably six, bearers should carry the stretcher (litter) at all times.
- Over rough terrain, eight carriers (six over smooth trail) should carry the litter for 15 minutes and then rest or rotate with other carriers.

Even when rescue help is requested (e.g., via cell phone), a detailed written note describing the situation and victim's condition should be completed. When without a cell phone, one or two members of the party can carry out a written request for help.

■ First Aid Kits

Most injuries and sudden illnesses do not require medical care. For all remote locations, it is a good idea to have useful supplies available for emergencies.

A first aid kit's supplies should be customized to include those items that are likely to be used on a regular basis, including nonprescription (over-the-counter) medications. Some medications lose their potency over time, especially after they have been opened; check expiration dates twice a year. Keep all medicines out of the reach of children. Read and follow all directions for proper medication use.

The following list contains useful first aid kit items. Change the list to meet the needs of situations that you are likely to encounter.

Item	Purpose
Micropore paper tape (1" and 2")	Covers blisters
Elastikon tape (2" and 4")	Covers wounds and blisters
Spenco 2nd Skin (1" and 3")	Covers wounds and blisters
Alcohol hand sanitizer gel (small bottle)	Cleans hands and the area around the wound (not inside wound)
Antibiotic ointment (Polysporin, Neosporin, Bacitracin, triple-antibiotic ointment)	Prevents skin infections that are associated with shallow wounds and makes nonstick dressings *(continued)*

Item	Purpose
Aloe vera gel (100% gel)	Apply to skin for sunburn or superficial frostbite.
Moleskin/molefoam	Apply over "hot spots" before blister formation. Several layers cut into a doughnut shape are useful for painful blisters.
Irrigation syringe (10 cc or 20 cc)	Provides pressure irrigation of wounds
Bandage strips (various sizes; also known as Band-Aids)	Covers minor wounds
Sterile gauze pads (2" x 2" and 4" x 4"; individually wrapped)	Covers wounds
Nonstick pads	Covers burns, blisters, and scrapes
Self-adhering roller bandage (2" to 4" wide; Kerlix, Kling)	Holds dressings in place
Sterile trauma pad (5" x 9", 8" x 10")	Covers large wounds
Elastic bandage (4" wide; Ace wrap)	Provides compression to reduce the swelling of joint injuries
Adhesive tape–various types available (e.g., athletic tape, hypoallergenic tape, waterproof tape)	Secures dressings and splints
Duct tape (very small roll)	Covers skin "hot spots" before blister formation, holds a dressing or splint, and has many other uses
Safety pins (2" long)	Creates sling from shirttail or sleeve, secures dressings, and drains blisters

(continued)

Item	Purpose
Pain and anti-inflammatory medication—for children, use acetaminophen (Tylenol); for adults, use aspirin or ibuprofen (Advil, Motrin).	Treats pain, fever, and swelling. Give only acetaminophen for children. Acetaminophen does not reduce swelling.
Decongestant tablets (e.g., Sudafed) Decongestant spray (e.g., Afrin, Neo-Synephrine)	Relieves nasal and upper respiratory congestion of viral colds, allergies, and sinus infections. Spray can be helpful in controlling nosebleeds.
Antihistamine (e.g., Benadryl)	Relieves allergy symptoms and treats poison ivy or oak itching and rash. It reduces nausea and motion sickness, causes drowsiness, and induces sleep.
Hydrocortisone cream, 1%	Soothes inflammation associated with insect bites and stings, poison ivy and oak, and other allergic skin rashes. It may be too weak for some conditions.
Calamine lotion (tends to be in large bottles and thus may not be practical to carry)	Anti-itch and drying agent for poison ivy or oak and skin rashes
Commercial sports drink packets (e.g., Gatorade)	Treats heat stress, dehydration, and "water intoxication" when too much water has been consumed and sodium has been depleted from body.
Sunscreen lotion (with at least SPF 15)	Prevents sunburn and windburn
Lip balm (with at least SPF 15)	Prevents sunburn and chapping of lips and soothes cold sores

(continued)

Item	Purpose
Insect repellent with DEET (< 30%)	Repels insects. For children, use no more than 10% DEET. Permethrin on clothes repels ticks.
Antacids tablets (e.g., Tums and Rolaids)	Treats heartburn and acid indigestion
Antidiarrheal tablets (e.g., Pepto-Bismol and Imodium A-D)	Treats diarrhea
Anticonstipation tablets (e.g., Metamucil)	Treats constipation
Scissors - various types available	Cut dressings, bandages, and clothing
Tweezers (angled tip)	Removes splinters and ticks
Thermometer, digital (75° F to 105° F)	Measures fever
SAM splint	Stabilizes broken bones and dislocations
Medical exam gloves	Protects against potentially infected blood and body fluids
Mouth-to-barrier device	Protects against potential infection during rescue breathing/CPR
Emergency blanket (e.g., state highway department trash bags; household polyethylene trash bags; "space blanket" made of Mylar, although may tear in wind)	Protects against body heat loss and weather (wind, rain, and snow)
Small notebook/pencil	Records information
Small first aid manual	Quick reference during an emergency and is used for learning first aid procedures

Basic Survival Kit: The Bare Essentials

Carry this kit whenever you are in remote areas.

Minimal Items	Purpose
One or two large, heavy-duty plastic bags (similar to state highway department trash bags), household polyethylene trash bags, or emergency blanket ("space blanket") made of Mylar, although it may tear in wind	Protects against weather (wind, rain, snow). Wear one trash bag by cutting hole in bottom of bag for head to fit through; use the second bag to cover legs.
Whistle*	Signal for help.
Signal mirror**	Signal for help.
Metal match with striker (magnesium)	Start a fire.
Waterproof match case containing windproof/waterproof matches	Start a fire.
Waterproof match case or empty film canister containing several cotton balls smeared with petroleum jelly (Vaseline)	Petroleum jelly is flammable. Make tinder using cotton balls smeared with petroleum jelly. When using, open the cotton ball to catch sparks from metal match.
Knife (multitool) and/or wire blade survival saw	Used for cutting
Food***	Provides calories and a psychological boost

* Whistle: A whistle is far superior to shouting. The whistle will carry for 0.5 to 2.0 miles or more in the wilderness, whereas your voice may only carry a few hundred yards. You will be able to signal for longer periods of time. Give three blasts in succession, repeated at intervals, to get attention. New high-tech whistles such as the "Storm" (from All-Weather Safety Whistle Co.) and the "Fox 40" (from Fox 40 International) and the smaller, more compact versions of these super whistles, the Windstorm and the Fox 40 Mini CMG, are much louder than police or referee whistles.

** Signal mirror: A mirror of 4 × 5 inches (standard U.S. Coast Guard size) or 3 × 5 inches is ideal, but the smaller 2 × 3 inch size also works well. Specially made glass and plastic signal mirrors are available. If you do not have a mirror, improvise using any piece of metal (polish it with fine sand or dirt), foil, or any shiny object. A mirror works even on overcast days and with moonlight, although with reduced range.

*** Food: Good items to carry include energy bars, candy bars, hard candy (e.g., lemon drops), powdered chocolate, dehydrated soup, or MREs (meals ready to eat). Discard any with soon-to-lapse expiration dates.

■ Finding Out What Is Wrong: Victim Assessment

A good victim assessment is essential to finding the problem to be treated and determining if medical care is needed. The saying, "find it; fix it," stresses that you cannot provide first aid unless you know what is wrong.

Check a victim systematically. Do this by performing these four steps:

1. Scene Size-Up
2. Primary Assessment

3. Secondary Assessment with three parts:
   A. Physical Exam
   B. Vital Signs
   C. SAMPLE History
4. Documentation

In most cases:

1. Take charge of the situation. You should have already made a decision about helping those in need of first aid. Identify yourself as a first aid provider to the victim and bystanders. If someone is already in charge, ask whether you can help.

2. Obtain permission (known as consent) from the victim to help. Consent is implied for an unresponsive victim, a responsive victim who remains silent and does not resist receiving first aid, and for children when a parent is not available.

3. Protect yourself from contact with blood and/or other body fluids by wearing disposable gloves and glasses, when available. A barrier device is recommended when giving breaths during CPR. If possible, wash your hands with soap and water, rubbing hands and fingers for at least 20 seconds, before providing care, and definitely wash your hands after giving first aid.

●●●●●●●●●●●●●●●●●●●●●

4. Most victims do not require a complete assessment (described below).

5. If you find a significant medical problem during a victim assessment, stop and immediately provide treatment.

6. Emergencies may require attracting the attention of rescuers. Yell for help or use a whistle to attract nearby bystanders. You may have to send another person(s) for help. Other means of seeking help include using a phone or a radio. Using the techniques found in the *Signaling for Help* section of this field guide can attract rescuers.

1. Scene Size-Up

As you approach the scene, ask yourself these questions:

A. **Is it safe for you, the victim(s), and any bystander(s)?** If the scene appears dangerous, stay away and seek help from trained rescuers. **DO NOT** try a rescue that you have not been trained for. You cannot help the victim if you also become a victim.

B. **How many people are involved?** There could be more than one victim, so look around and ask about others. If there are two or more victims, go to the quiet, motionless victim(s) first.

C. **What is wrong?** Form a first impression of the victim by asking yourself if he/she is: (1) injured or ill,

(2) responsive or unresponsive, (3) breathing normally, or (4) bleeding severely.

D. How was the victim injured or how did the victim become ill? Look for clues about what caused the injury or the nature of the illness.

2. Primary Assessment

The purpose of the primary assessment is to identify and treat ("find it; fix it") life-threatening problems requiring immediate care. If you find a life-threatening problem, stop and treat it before continuing through the assessment. Victims fall into one of two types: unresponsive or responsive.

For an alert, responsive victim: RAP-ABC-DE

You are more likely to see this type of victim. Use **RAP-ABC-DE** to recall the sequence of what to do.

R – Check **responsiveness** by making eye contact, introducing yourself, and asking if you can help. The victim may give permission for you to help by saying yes or nodding the head.

A – **Ask** the victim, "What happened?" and "Where do you hurt?" (known as the chief complaint). If the victim appears to be severely injured or ill, **ask** another person(s) to go or to call for help by using a cell phone, satellite phone, or radio.

P – Position victim in a comfortable position (such as lying down or leaning against a stable object).

A – Maintain open **airway**. A talking victim has an open airway.

B – Monitor **breathing**—are there abnormal breathing sounds (such as wheezing, gurgling, snoring)? This field guide covers breathing problems in several other sections.

C – Check **circulation**—is there severe bleeding (blood spurting or rapidly flowing from a wound)? For how to control bleeding, refer to the *Bleeding and Wound Care* section of this field guide.

Continue the assessment. See the following section for completing the **D** and **E** parts of the assessment.

For a motionless, unresponsive victim: RAB-CAB-DE

These steps resemble the same steps for starting cardiopulmonary resuscitation (CPR)—**RAB-CAB-DE**—although most unresponsive victims do not need CPR.

R – Check **responsiveness** by tapping victim's shoulder and shouting "Are you OK?" Check for breathing and gasping.

A – If there is no response, **activate** EMS by asking another person(s) to go or call for help by using a cell phone, satellite phone, or radio.

B – **Breathing?** With the person face up on a flat, firm surface, observe the person's chest for movement (rise and fall); take 5–10 seconds. If the victim is breathing and no spinal injury is suspected, place on his/her side and check for severe bleeding.

C – If the victim is not breathing or only gasping, give CPR starting with 30 **chest compressions**—push hard; push fast. Use the same beat as the Bee Gee's song, "Stayin' Alive."

A – Open **airway** by tilting head back and lifting chin to move the tongue away from the back of the throat. Do this for all victims, even when spinal injury is suspected.

B – Give two **breaths** (each lasting 1 second and making the chest rise).

Continue cycles of 30 compressions and 2 rescue breaths until an AED arrives, another trained person takes over, you are too exhausted to continue, or the victim revives. If you do not know CPR, give continuous chest compressions without breaths.

For an unresponsive, normal-breathing victim, maintain an open airway, monitor breathing, and continue the assessment.

D and E for All Victims

D – **Disability**. Tell the alert victim not to move. Whenever you suspect a head or spinal injury, have a bystander stabilize the victim's head by holding it still. A more decisive check for spinal injuries happens later during the Physical Exam, while checking the arms and legs. Refer to the *Head Injuries* and *Spinal Cord Injury* sections in this field guide.

E – **Environment** and **Expose** injuries. Prolonged exposure to extreme temperatures (cold and heat) can threaten life. Such conditions may point to the cause of the victim's problem.

Clothing may have to be removed down to the skin to check and treat an injury. If you need to remove clothing, explain what you intend to do and why to the victim and bystanders. Remove only as much clothing as necessary, try to maintain privacy, and prevent exposure to cold.

3. Secondary Assessment

This assessment consists of three parts: Physical Exam, Vital Signs, and SAMPLE History.

A. Physical Exam (Hands-On Exam)

Most victims require only a physical exam of the body area localized by the chief complaint; a full body physical exam (described below) is not needed. Just as in the Primary Assessment, any life-threatening injuries should be immediately treated before continuing through an assessment. Otherwise, complete the entire Secondary Assessment before treating an injury.

Check a part of the body by looking and gently feeling for **DOTS**:

D: Deformity—abnormal shape of the body part (compare it against the opposite uninjured part). Deformities occur when bones are broken or joints are dislocated.

O: Open wounds—the skin is broken and there is bleeding.

T: Tenderness—sensitivity, discomfort, or pain when touched.

S: Swelling—area looks larger than usual. This is caused by excess fluid in the tissue. Compare one side of the body with the other side (for example, if an ankle appears swollen, compare it with the uninjured one).

This is a full-body, head-to-toe, hands-on assessment on an alert and awake victim. If you suspect a spinal injury, stabilize the head and neck against movement. Start looking and feeling at the head and work your way toward the toes. Explain what you will be doing and **DO NOT** be afraid of touching the victim after you have gained his/her permission (consent) to help. When looking and gently feeling for DOTS on an unresponsive victim, he/she will not be able to tell you about the "T" for tenderness.

1. **Head**–check for DOTS, and assess skin condition for temperature, color, and moisture. Look for eye damage, fluid in the ears and nose, and objects and fluid in the mouth.
2. **Neck**–check for DOTS; firmly push on the bony part of the spine from the bottom of the skull to the top of the shoulders for tenderness and deformity. Look for a medical identification tag or necklace.
3. **Shoulders**–check for DOTS, including the collarbone.

4. **Chest**–check for DOTS; gently squeeze the chest inward and ask if doing so is painful.
5. **Abdomen**–check for DOTS; gently push downward on all four of the abdominal quadrants using the navel as the central point.
6. **Pelvis**–gently press downward followed by a gentle squeeze inward on the hip bones (iliac crests).
7. **Genitals**–check only if an injury is suspected.
8. **Legs**–check for DOTS from the groin to the toes. Check for a spinal injury by (a) pinching the end of several toes without allowing victim to see his/her feet and asking which toe is being pinched, (b) having the victim wiggle the toes, and (c) having the victim push his/her feet against your hand.
9. **Arms**–check for DOTS from the armpit to the fingers. Check for a spinal injury by (a) pinching the end of several fingers without allowing victim to see the fingers and asking which finger is being pinched, (b) having the victim wiggle fingers, and (c) having the victim squeeze your hand with each hand. Look for a medical identification bracelet around a wrist.
10. **Back**–Combine this step with what was found while checking the legs and arms. If no spinal injury is suspected, check the back for DOTS and firmly push on the spine's bony parts from the shoulders to the pelvis for tenderness and/or deformity.

If a spinal injury is suspected, use others to help roll the victim onto his/her side, keeping his/her nose and navel pointing in the same direction. **DO NOT** twist the torso or neck. Check for DOTS and firmly push spine's bony parts from the shoulders to the pelvis, checking for tenderness and/or deformity.

Medical Identification Tag

A medical identification tag (such as on a bracelet or necklace) contains the wearer's medical problem(s) and a 24-hour telephone number. The tag can sometimes help identify what is wrong with the victim. If looking in a wallet or a purse (note: this might be illegal in some states) for medical identification, always have another person present to avoid later accusations should money or credit cards be missing.

B. Vital Signs

Vital signs can show a victim's overall condition rather than a specific problem. They show what is going on inside the body. Taking vital signs at 15 to 20 minute intervals over time can indicate whether the victim is getting better, getting worse, or remaining about the same. The vital signs include: level of responsiveness, heart rate, breathing rate, and skin condition.

Level of Responsiveness: AVPU Scale

A victim's level of responsiveness can range from fully responsive (conscious) to unresponsive (unconscious). The four-level AVPU scale describes the victim's responsiveness. The scale indicates how the brain is doing.

AVPU Scale

A	**Alert** and aware (eyes open; can answer questions clearly; knows name and where he/she is)
V	Responds to **Voice** in some way when spoken to (attempts to speak, groans, or moves)
P	Responds to **Pain** (responds to pinching of skin next to the neck above the collarbone—when pinching, **DO NOT** injure the victim)
U	**Unresponsive** (no response to Voice or Pain)

Heart Rate (HR)

The heart rate (also known as the pulse rate) is the number of heartbeats per minute. The normal rate for an adult at rest is between 60 and 100 beats per minute. An exception is an athlete in good health with a normal resting heart rate between 40 and 50 beats per minute. Be concerned about the adult whose heart rate stays above 100 or below 60 beats per minute. If the heart rate is taken several times and he/she maintains it above 120 beats or below 50 beats per minute, something may be seriously wrong that requires medical care.

Measure the heart rate by placing the flat part of the ends of your index and middle fingers two inches above the base of the thumb on the inside of the wrist (known as the radial pulse site). **DO NOT** use your thumb, because you might feel your own pulse. Count the beats for 30 seconds, then multiply by two to get the heart rate in beats per minute.

A heartbeat felt at the wrist (radial pulse) indicates that enough blood pressure exists to saturate all the body tissues with oxygenated blood.

Breathing Rate (BR)

One breath consists of one inhalation and one exhalation. The breathing rate (also known as the respiration rate) is the number of breaths taken in one minute. The normal breathing rate of an adult at rest is 12 to 20 breaths per minute. A rate less than 8 or greater than 24 is abnormal and may indicate a problem requiring supplemental oxygen.

Count the breathing rate by watching the victim's chest rise and fall for 30 seconds, counting each time the victim inhales and then multiplying this number by two. Some victims may deliberately change their breathing rate if they know you are counting them. Try to count the breathing without the victim's knowledge by pretending to be taking the heart rate.

Abnormal sounds such as gurgling, crowing, wheezing, snoring, or gasping can indicate a medical problem.

Skin Condition: Color, Temperature, and Moisture

Skin color, especially in light-skinned people, reflects the circulation under the skin as well as oxygen status. For those with dark complexions, changes might not be readily apparent but can be assessed in all people by the appearance of the nail beds, the inside of the lips, and/or under the eyelids.

Get a rough idea of skin temperature by putting the inside of your wrist or the back of your hand on the victim's forehead to determine whether the temperature is elevated or decreased. If unsure, try comparing the victim's temperature with a known healthy person. Dry skin is normal. Skin that is wet, moist (unless the victim has been sweating or in water), or excessively dry and hot suggests a problem.

C. SAMPLE History

A SAMPLE history helps identify what is wrong. Often the victim can tell you, but if he/she cannot, the information may be obtained from family, friends, bystanders, or a medical identification tag.

S = Symptoms	"What is wrong? Where do you hurt?" (known as the chief complaint)
A = Allergies	"Are you allergic to anything?"
M = Medications	"Are you taking any medications? What are they for? When were they last taken?"

P = **P**ertinent past history	"Have you had this problem before? Do you have other medical problems?"
L = **L**ast intake and output	"When did you last eat or drink anything? What was it? How much? When was the last time you urinated or defecated? Were they normal?"
E = **E**vents leading up to the injury or illness	Injury: "How did you get hurt?" Illness: "What led to this problem?"

For a chief complaint involving an illness, you cannot diagnose the exact cause of the illness. Instead, determine if it is serious enough to require medical care.

4. Documentation

For medical and legal reasons, a report should be written as soon as possible, but this should not interfere with a victim's treatment. The following SOAP method enables you to document the incident quickly and accurately. Without detracting from the treatment, taking photos as soon as possible of the scene and the injury may be helpful for legal reasons or later medical care.

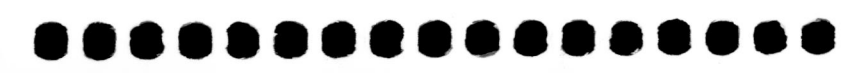

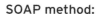

SOAP method:

S = Subjective	What did you find in the SAMPLE history?
O = Objective	What did you find during the scene size-up, primary assessment, vital signs, and physical exam?
A = Assessment	What do you think was wrong?
P = Plan	What are you going to do for each problem?

SOAP Note (example)

Victim Name: _____

Date & Time of Incident: _____

Age: _____ Gender: M or F   Location: _____

Weather: _____

S - Subjective: What did the victim tell you? (based upon SAMPLE history)

S = Symptoms/chief complaint(s):	1.
	2.
	3.
A = Allergies:	
M = Medications:	
P = Pertinent medical history:	
L = Last oral intake:	
E = Events leading:	

O - Objective: What did you observe?

Physical exam (includes DOTS)

Head:	Abdomen:
Eyes, ears, nose, mouth:	Pelvis:
Neck:	Extremities:
Shoulders:	Back:
Chest:	Medical ID tag:

Vital Signs

Date/Time	AVPU level	Heart rate	Breathing rate	Skin condition

A - Assessment: What do you think is wrong?

1.		3.	
2.		4.	

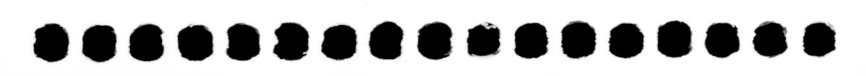

P – Plan: What are you going to do for each of the problems in Assessment section?

First Aid given for each problem	Medical care needed?	Evacuate? If yes, how?
1.		
2.		
3.		
4.		

Verbal First Aid: What to Say to a Victim

Avoid negative statements that may add to victim's distress, fear, and pain. Use simple words to create confidence, comfort, and cooperation.

1. Your first words to a victim are very important.
2. **DO NOT** ask unnecessary questions (e.g., "What did you do?") unless it aids treatment or satisfies the victim's need to talk.
3. Make no negative value judgments.
4. Link a suggestion that you want the injured person to accept with a statement he or she cannot deny (e.g., "That leg is probably hurting, but we'll soon make you comfortable").

5. Tears and/or laughter can be normal—tell the injured person this if such responses seem to make him or her feel embarrassed or guilty.

6. Stress the positive, but be realistic (e.g., instead of "You will not have any pain," say "You will feel better").

7. **DO NOT** deny the obvious (e.g., instead of saying, "There is nothing wrong," say, "You've had quite a fall and probably don't feel too good, but we're going to look after you; you'll soon be feeling better").

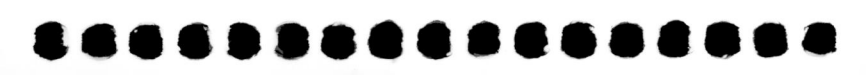

A-Z of Injuries and Sudden Illnesses

■ Abdominal Complaints

Abdominal Pain

There are many possible causes of abdominal pain, some not so serious and some life threatening. Some can be serious enough to require immediate evacuation for medical care. Illnesses affecting the abdomen have two things in common: they are very painful, and even skilled physicians may have trouble pinpointing an exact cause. It is impractical for a first aid provider to distinguish among the many causes of abdominal pain because first aid will usually be similar regardless of the cause.

What to Do

1. Give water or clear fluids such as sports drinks or clear soups (no alcohol or caffeine). Have victim slowly sip the fluids. Avoid solid foods. Later, give clear soups and bland foods (e.g., toast, oatmeal).

2. Give victim an antacid (e.g., Tums, Rolaids, Pepto-Bismol). If these fail, try a medication that helps stop stomach acid secretion (e.g., Tagamet and Pepcid AC). If these fail, seek medical advice.

3. If practical, place a hot-water bottle against the victim's abdomen, or have the victim soak in a warm bath.

4. Be prepared for vomiting.

5. Have the victim lie down with knees bent. Seek medical help if any of these apply:

   - Pain is constant for more than 6 hours.
   - The victim is unable to eat or drink fluids.
   - The victim is or may be pregnant.
   - Significant recent abdominal injury exists.
   - The abdomen is rigid and painful.
   - After pressing your fingers on victim's abdomen and suddenly releasing it, more pain occurs.
   - There is bloody, blood stained, or black stool.
   - The victim has a high fever.
   - Pain began around the navel (belly button) and later moved to the lower right abdomen. This is a sign of appendicitis.

Nausea and Vomiting

Vomiting and nausea often occur with conditions such as acute mountain sickness, motion sickness, brain injury, intestinal viruses, eating or drinking too much, and emotional distress.

What to Do

1. Give water or clear fluids such as sports drinks or clear soups (no alcohol or caffeine). Have victim slowly sip the fluids. Avoid solid foods. Later, give clear soups and bland foods (e.g., toast, crackers, and oatmeal).
2. Rest and avoid exertion until the victim is able to eat solid foods easily.
3. Be prepared for vomiting.
4. Seek medical help if any of these apply:

   - Blood or brown, grainy material appears in vomit.
   - Constant abdominal pain exists.
   - Victim faints when standing.
   - Victim is unable to keep fluids down for more than 24 hours.
   - Heavy or forceful vomiting occurs.
   - Victim suffered an abdominal injury.
   - Vomiting follows a recent head injury.

Diarrhea

Diarrhea is the frequent (usually more than four times a day) passage of loose, watery, or unformed stools. Some experts say to let diarrhea run its course because bacteria or parasites are expelled and are not trapped in the intestines.

What to Do

1. Give water or clear fluids such as sports drinks or clear soups (no alcohol or caffeine). Have the victim slowly sip the fluids. Avoid solid foods. Later, give clear soups and bland foods (e.g., toast, crackers, oatmeal).
2. Give Pepto-Bismol (follow the label directions). It can turn the stool and tongue black. Those who are sensitive to aspirin and children under 12 should not use it. If the victim must be in control of his or her stools, Imodium A-D can reduce the movement of food through the intestines.
3. Seek medical help if any of these apply:
   - Blood in stools that may appear black (keep in mind that Pepto-Bismol can cause black stools)
   - No improvement after 24 hours
   - Fever
   - Severe, constant abdominal pain
   - Severe dehydration

Constipation

Constipation is the passage of hard, dry stools occurring fewer than three times a week.

What to Do

1. Make sure the victim drinks plenty of fluids (8 to 10 eight-ounce glasses daily).

2. Have the victim eat fiber (fresh or dried fruits, vegetables, or bran). Over-the-counter fiber products (e.g., Metamucil or Citrucel) can be used (follow label directions). **DO NOT** give a laxative.

3. Encourage the victim to remain active.

4. If no improvement occurs, try milk of magnesia or caffeine.

5. Seek medical help if any of these apply:

- Severe abdominal pain
- Visibly swollen abdomen accompanied by pain
- Fever
- Vomiting

■ Abdominal Injuries

What to Look for	What to Do
Penetrating object	**DO NOT** remove a penetrating object. Stabilize the object against movement. **DO NOT** give the victim anything to eat or drink. Seek medical help.
Protruding organs	**DO NOT** try to push protruding organs back into the abdomen. **DO NOT** touch organs. Cover them with a moist, clean dressing. **DO NOT** give the victim anything to eat or drink. Seek medical help.

(continued)

What to Look for	What to Do
Hard blow to abdomen	Roll the victim on one side and expect vomiting. **DO NOT** give the victim anything to eat or drink. Seek medical help.

■ Alcohol and Drug Emergencies

Alcohol Intoxication

What to Look for	What to Do
· Odor of alcohol · Unsteady, staggering gait · Slurred speech and inability to carry on a conversation · Nausea and vomiting · Flushed face	1. Monitor breathing. 2. Check for injuries. 3. Keep victim on his/her side.

Drugs

Drugs are classified according to their effects on the user.

What to Look for	What to Do
· **Uppers** stimulate the central nervous system. Examples are amphetamines and cocaine.	1. Monitor breathing. *(continued)*

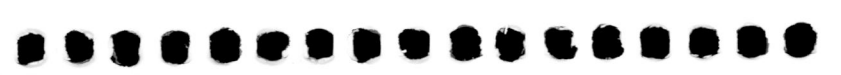

What to Look for	What to Do
• **Downers** depress the central nervous system. Examples are barbiturates, tranquilizers, marijuana, and narcotics. • **Hallucinogens** alter the senses (e.g., vision). Examples are LSD, mescaline, peyote, and PCP (angel dust). Marijuana also has some hallucinogenic capabilities. • **Volatile chemicals** usually are inhaled and can seriously damage many body organs. Examples are paint solvents, gasoline, and spray paint.	2. Check for injuries. 3. Keep victim on his/her side. 4. Seek medical help.

Warning

- **DO NOT** let an intoxicated or drugged person sleep on his or her back.
- **DO NOT** leave an intoxicated or drugged person alone.
- **DO NOT** try to handle a violent person by yourself—find a safe place, and call law enforcement officials.

■ Allergic Reactions (Severe)

Severe reactions to medications, food and food additives, insect stings, and plant pollen can be life threatening (called anaphylaxis).

What to Look for

- Warm feeling followed by intense itching
- Skin flushes; face may swell
- Sneezing, coughing, wheezing
- Shortness of breath
- Tightness and swelling in the throat
- Tightness in the chest
- Increased heart rate
- Swelling of tongue, mouth, nose
- Blueness around lips and mouth
- Dizziness
- Nausea and vomiting

What to Do

1. Monitor breathing.
2. If the victim has his/her own physician-prescribed epinephrine, help the victim use it. Inject at mid-thigh (can be given through clothing). About 25% to 35% require a second dose.
3. If the victim can swallow, give antihistamine (Benadryl)—it is not lifesaving because it takes too long to work, but can prevent further reactions.
4. Seek medical help ASAP.

■ Altitude Illnesses

Going above 8,000 feet (2,500 meters) can produce one of several types of altitude illnesses. Altitude illnesses are caused by a prolonged lack of oxygen in the blood and tissues due to low air pressure at higher elevations. **Figure 2**

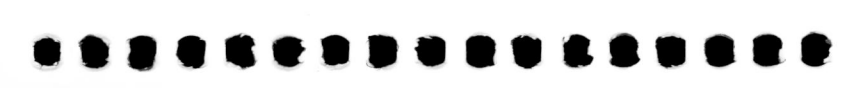

Acute Mountain Sickness (AMS)	High-Altitude Cerebral Edema (HACE)—fluid collects in brain, causing it to swell	High-Altitude Pulmonary Edema (HAPE)—fluid collects in lungs
What to Look for Headache plus one or more of the following: · Fatigue · Dizziness · Sleep disturbance · Nausea with or without vomiting · Loss of appetite	**What to Look for** Severe headache, usually throbbing, plus one or more of the following: · Extreme fatigue · Cannot walk straight · Dizziness · Sleep disturbance · Nausea/vomiting · Altered mental status	**What to Look for** · Shortness of breath · Dry cough; later has frothy pink sputum · Mild chest pain · Weakness · Sleep disturbance · Rapid heart rate (>100 beats per minute when resting) · Crackling or gurgling breath sounds
What to Do 1. Stop ascending (going up), rest, and wait for symptoms to improve (12 hours to several days). If symptoms do not improve, descend (go down) until symptoms decrease, usually 1,000–3,000 feet (300–1,000 meters). Victim should not go down alone.	**What to Do** 1. Rapidly descend (go down) until symptoms decrease, usually 1,000–3,000 feet (300–1,000 meters). Victim should not go down alone. 2. Give the victim fluids.	**What to Do** 1. Rapidly descend (go down) until symptoms decrease, usually 1,000–3,000 feet (300–1,000 meters). Victim should not go down alone. 2. If available and you are trained, give high-flow supplemental oxygen. *(continued)*

2. Have victim self-administer pain medication for headache and anti-emetics for nausea/vomiting relief. 3. If available and you are trained, give high-flow supplemental oxygen. 4. Give the victim fluids.	3. If descent is not immediately possible: • Give high-flow supplemental oxygen, if available and you are trained, or • Use portable hyperbaric chamber, if available and you are trained. **DO NOT** delay descent. 4. Seek medical help ASAP.	3. If available and you are trained, use portable hyperbaric chamber if descent is not immediately possible. **DO NOT** delay descent. 4. Seek medical help ASAP.

Other Altitude-Related Illnesses

Pharyngitis and Bronchitis

Because of dry air, a sore throat and coughing may develop. The victim should drink fluids, have antibiotic ointment applied in the nose, and suck hard candy or throat lozenges. For dry coughing, give a cough medicine (e.g., Robitussin DM).

Peripheral Edema

Swelling of hands, ankles, and/or face (around eyes) may appear at higher altitudes. If possible, raise the victim's arms and/or legs. After descending or with acclimatization to higher altitudes, the swelling usually diminishes. Descend if signs of more serious altitude illnesses appear.

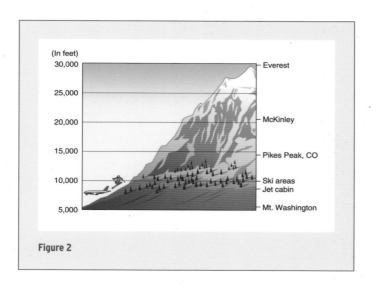

(In feet)

- Everest
- McKinley
- Pikes Peak, CO
- Ski areas
- Jet cabin
- Mt. Washington

Figure 2

■ Arthropod Bites and Stings

Arthropods—including scorpions, spiders, centipedes, and ticks—are invertebrates with jointed legs and segmented bodies. Stinging insects cause more deaths than do venomous snakes. **Figures 3-6**

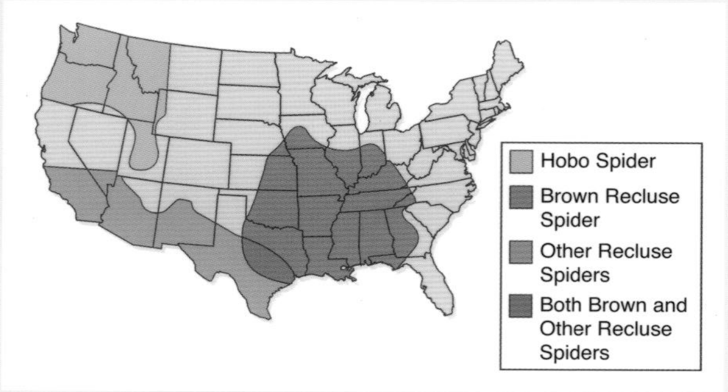

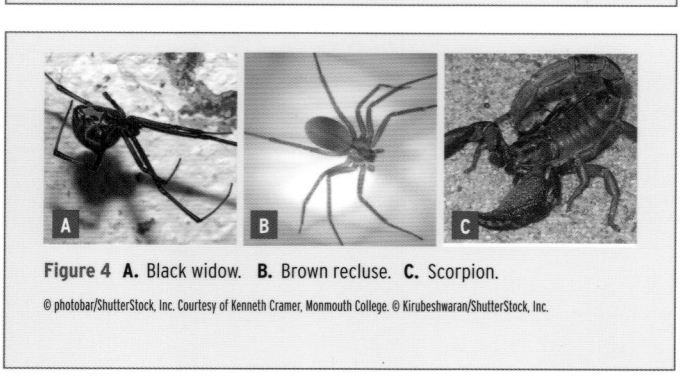

Figure 3

Figure 4 A. Black widow. **B.** Brown recluse. **C.** Scorpion.

© photobar/ShutterStock, Inc. Courtesy of Kenneth Cramer, Monmouth College. © Kirubeshwaran/ShutterStock, Inc.

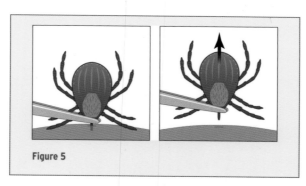

Figure 5

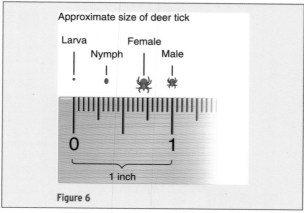

Approximate size of deer tick

Larva
Nymph
Female
Male

1 inch

Figure 6

Arthropod	What to Look for	What to Do
Stinging insects · Honeybee · Bumblebee · Hornet · Yellow jacket · Wasp · Fire ants Those who have had a previous severe reaction should wear a medical alert ID tag and carry a physician-prescribed epinephrine kit.	· Usual reactions: instant pain, redness, itching. · Worrisome reactions: hives, swollen lips/tongue, "tickle" in throat, wheezing. · Life-threatening reactions: blue/gray skin color, seizures, unresponsiveness, inability to breathe because of swollen vocal cords. · About 60% to 80% of anaphylactic deaths are caused by victim's inability to breathe because of swollen airway passages.	1. Look for a stinger, and if found, remove it as soon as possible (e.g., brush off with your hand or scrape it with a fingernail). **DO NOT** use tweezers. Only bees leave their stinger embedded. 2. Wash with soap and water. 3. Apply cold to the area. Baking soda paste may help except for wasp stings. 4. Give pain medication. Apply hydrocortisone cream (1%) and give antihistamine (Benadryl). 5. For a severe allergic reaction, help victim self-administer epinephrine.

(continued)

Arthropod	What to Look for	What to Do
Widow spider bites Best known as the black widow, but the term "black widow" is inaccurate because only three of the five species of widow spiders are black; the others are brown and gray. Only adult females bite. They have a shiny, black abdomen with a red or yellow spot that is often in shape of hourglass, or white spots or bands on the abdomen.	· May feel sharp pinprick followed by dull, numbing pain · Two small fang marks seen as tiny red spots · Severe abdominal pain (bites on arm can produce severe chest pain, thus mimicking a heart attack) · Headache, chills, fever, heavy sweating, nausea, and vomiting · Most victims never see the spider.	1. Clean with soap and water. 2. Apply cold to the area. 3. Give pain medication. 4. Seek medical help ASAP. *(continued)*

Arthropod	What to Look for	What to Do
Fiddle back spider bites Also known as brown recluse spider, violin spider, and brown spider.	• Mild to severe pain occurs within 2 to 8 hours. • A blister develops within 48 to 72 hours, becomes red, and bursts. It takes on a "bull's-eye" appearance. • Nausea, vomiting, headache, and fever	Same as for black widow spider. If wound becomes infected, apply antibiotic ointment under sterile dressing.
Hobo spider bites Also known as the aggressive house spider.	Same as for fiddle back spiders.	Same as for fiddle back spiders.
Tarantula spider bites They bite only when vigorously provoked or roughly handled. They can flick their hairs onto a person's skin.	• Pain varies from mild to severe throbbing lasting up to 1 hour.	Same as for black widow spider. For hairs in the skin, remove with sticky tape, wash with soap and water, apply hydrocortisone cream (1%), and give antihistamine and pain medication.

(continued)

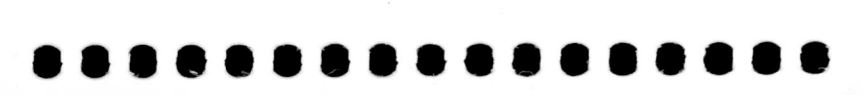

Arthropod	What to Look for	What to Do
Scorpion stings In the United States, only the bark scorpion found in Arizona is potentially deadly–it is active from May through August.	• Burning pain • Numbness or tingling occurs later.	1. Monitor breathing. 2. Wash with soap and water. 3. Apply cold to the area. 4. Give pain medication. 5. Apply dressing. 6. Seek medical help for severe reactions.
Centipede bites Do not confuse with millipedes, which cannot inject venom but can irritate the skin.	• Burning pain • Inflammation • Mild swelling of lymph nodes	Most bites will get better without treatment. 1. Clean the wound with soap and water. 2. Apply cold. 3. Give pain medication. 4. If symptoms persist, give antihistamine (Benadryl) or apply hydrocortisone cream (1%) on the bite site. 5. Seek medical help for severe reactions. *(continued)*

Arthropod	What to Look for	What to Do
Embedded tick Most ticks are harmless, but can carry diseases (i.e., Lyme disease, Rocky Mountain spotted fever, Colorado tick fever, Tularemia, etc.). If a tick is carrying a disease, the longer it stays embedded, the greater the chance of the disease will be transmitted.	• No pain initially exists, and the tick can go unnoticed for days without detection. • Red area around tick means it has punctured skin and is feeding on victim's blood. • If engorged with blood, it means there is an increased risk of disease transmission. • May cause rash, fever, and chills. • The bite varies from a small bump to extensive swelling and ulcer.	Ticks are difficult to remove. Partial removal can lead to infection. 1. Use tweezers or a tick removal tool. Grasp the tick close to the skin and pull up, gently tenting the skin. Hold tension until the tick releases. **DO NOT** jerk or twist the tick. If the head is embedded in the skin, remove as you would a splinter. 2. Wash the area with soap and water. 3. Apply cold to the area. 4. If tick was engorged, seek medical advice. If traveling in "tick country," consult with a physician for advice before the trip. 5. Watch for signs of infection such as headache, fever, or rash appearing 3 to 30 days after the tick bite. If symptoms appear, seek medical advice.

(continued)

Arthropod	What to Look for	What to Do
		Cautions about removing an embedded tick: • **DO NOT** use a hot match, fingernail polish, alcohol, petroleum jelly, or gasoline.
Chigger mite bites Bites can number in the hundreds.	• Severe itching occurs after several hours. • Small red welts appear. • Skin infection can result.	1. Wash with soap and water and rinse several times. 2. Apply cold to the area. 3. Apply hydrocortisone cream (1%) or calamine lotion. 4. Give antihistamine (Benadryl). Effectiveness of applying clear nail polish is questionable.
Mosquito bites Human breath (contains carbon dioxide) and sweat attract mosquitoes.	• Itching • Mild swelling	1. Wash the affected area with soap and water. 2. Apply cold. 3. Apply calamine lotion or hydrocortisone cream (1%) to decrease itching.

(continued)

■ Asthma

Asthma is a lung condition that narrows the airway (tubes that carry air into and out of the lungs). The episodes can be occasional or often. Between episodes, the person has no trouble breathing. Asthma varies from one person to another, with symptoms ranging from mild to severe, and can be life threatening.

Arthropod	What to Look for	What to Do
Fleas	Itching • Multiple bites—termed "breakfast, lunch, and dinner"—are common.	1. Apply cold. 2. Apply hydrocortisone cream (1%). 3. Give an antihistamine. 4. For a victim of numerous stings or a delayed allergic reaction, an antihistamine (Benadryl) every 6 hours or a physician-prescribed cortisone might be helpful.

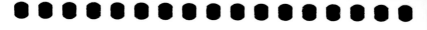

What to Look for

- Excessive coughing
- Wheezing (whistling or squeaky sound during breathing)
- Chest tightness
- Shortness of breath
- Sitting in tripod position (leaning forward with hands on knees or other support, trying to breathe)
- Inability to speak in complete sentences without stopping to breathe
- Nostrils flaring with each breath
- Fast breath and heart rates

What to Do

1. Place the victim in an upright sitting position, leaning slightly forward.
2. Monitor breathing.
3. Ask the victim about any asthma medication he/she uses. Most asthmatics usually have a doctor-prescribed quick-relief ("rescue") inhaler.
4. Help the victim use the quick-relief inhaler:
   a. Shake the inhaler vigorously several times, remove the cap, and apply the spacer, if available.
   b. Holding the inhaler upright, tell the victim to place his/her lips around the inhaler or spacer.
   c. As the victim breathes in slowly and deeply, depress the inhaler to release the medication.
   d. If using a spacer, press down on the inhaler and then wait 5 seconds before breathing in.
   e. Tell the victim to hold his/her breath for at least 10 seconds and to breathe out slowly.
   f. A second dose may be given in 30 to 60 seconds.
5. Seek medical help if:
   a. There is no improvement after using the medication.
   b. Repeated attacks occur.
   c. There is a severe and prolonged attack.

B

■ Bleeding and Wound Care

Bleeding Control

1. Expose the bleeding wound.

2. Avoid contact with blood by putting on disposable medical exam gloves. If gloves are unavailable, use a plastic bag, extra dressings, clean cloths, or have the victim apply pressure with his/her own hand, if possible.

3. Stop the bleeding by placing a sterile dressing or clean cloth over the wound and pushing on the wound. This technique stops most bleeding. If bleeding does not stop in 10 minutes, press harder over a wider area for another 10 minutes. For a gaping wound, pack the wound with a sterile dressing. **Figure 7**

Tourniquet Use

Consider using a tourniquet only if severe bleeding (i.e., spurting or flowing) from an arm or leg cannot be stopped by applying pressure to the wound.

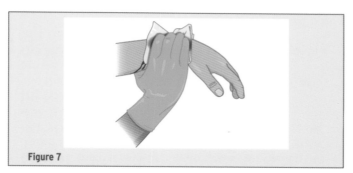

Figure 7

Hemostatic Dressing Use

When direct pressure is not effective, a tourniquet (TQ) is not available, a TQ is not effective, or a TQ cannot be applied (i.e., abdomen, back, chest), apply a hemostatic dressing in combination with direct pressure.

a. While making a tourniquet, continue applying pressure over the wound.

b. Make a tourniquet from a triangle bandage, neckerchief, wide roller bandage, or similar cloth into a long band about 3 to 4 inches wide and several layers thick. **DO NOT** use narrow materials (i.e., wire, rope, or cord), which could cut into the skin.

c. Wrap the band around the arm or leg twice, placing it about 2 inches above the wound (between the wound and the heart).

d.   Tie the ends together over the wound.

e.   Place a short (6 to 8 inches) stick or similar object on the knot and then tie another knot over the stick (a square knot is best).

f.   Twist the stick as you would a handle until bleeding stops. If a heartbeat can be felt at the wrist (for arm injuries) or behind the inside ankle knob (for a leg injury), the tourniquet is too loose. Secure the stick in place with another cloth band or tape to maintain the pressure.

g.   Write "TQ" (for tourniquet) and the exact time it was applied on a piece of adhesive tape and stick it to the victim's forehead. You could write this directly onto the victim's forehead skin if there is no tape available.

When using a tourniquet:

- **DO NOT** apply it anywhere except on an arm or leg—it does not work on the torso, head, neck, armpit, or groin.
- **DO NOT** apply it over any joint, but keep it close to the wound as possible.
- **DO NOT** use narrow materials.
- Use wide padding under the tourniquet, if possible, to protect the tissues and help apply compression.
- **DO NOT** cover a tourniquet—leave it in view unless in a cold environment.

- **DO NOT** release a tourniquet unless medical care is more than 1 hour away. In this situation, **DO NOT** take it off; instead, release the tourniquet every 2 hours to quickly see if the bleeding has stopped or slowed to the point that a pressure bandage over the wound would be sufficient. While long-term tourniquet use may result in an amputation, it is better than death due to blood loss.

Wound Care

1. Clean the wound (this may restart bleeding):
   a. For a shallow wound:
      - Wash inside and around the wound with soap and water.
      - Flush the inside of the wound with pressurized water that is clean enough to drink. This means using water from a faucet or an irrigation syringe. If using an irrigation syringe, flush 0.75 to 1 cup of water through the wound. Using a plastic bag with a small hole cut in it may be helpful. Pouring, soaking, or using a bulb syringe does not provide enough pressure to be effective but may be all that is available.
      - Cover the wound with a thin layer of an over-the-counter antibiotic ointment (e.g., Neosporin

or Polysporin). **DO NOT** use thiomersal
(Merthiolate), merbromin (Mercurochrome), or
hydrogen peroxide as these are toxic to the tissues.

b. For a wound with a high risk for infection (e.g., animal
bite, very dirty or ragged wound, puncture wound),
clean as best you can. Seek medical help ASAP.

2. Cover shallow and high-risk wounds with a sterile
dressing. Close small, clean wounds with tape or
"butterfly" strips if the edges can be easily pulled together.
Pack high-risk wounds with gauze dressings held in place
by a bandage.

3. Seek medical help to:

- Clean wounds at high risk for infection.
- Close wide and gaping open wounds or if an
  underlying structure (e.g., tendon, nerve) is injured.
- Receive a tetanus booster, if necessary.

When possible, scrub hands vigorously with soap and water
before and after giving help. If water is unavailable, use an
alcohol hand sanitizer gel.

Infected Wound

Any wound, large or small, can become infected. Proper
cleaning can help prevent infections.

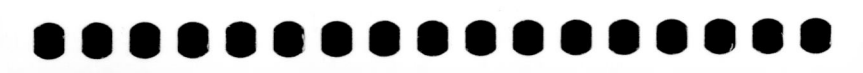

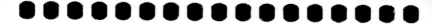

What to Look for	What to Do
• Swelling and redness around wound • Feels warmer than surrounding area • Throbbing pain • Pus discharge • Fever • Swelling of lymph nodes • One or more red streaks leading from the wound toward the heart; this is a serious sign that the infection is spreading.	1. Soak the wound in warm water, or apply warm, wet packs over the infected wound. Separate the wound edges to allow pus to escape. 2. Apply an antibiotic ointment. 3. Change the dressings several times a day. 4. Give pain medication. 5. Seek medical help if the wound becomes worse.

Blood Under a Nail

What to Look for	What to Do
A fingernail or toenail has been crushed or smashed, causing the victim unbearable pain because blood collects under the nail.	1. Relieve pressure under the injured nail by using one of the following methods: • Use the eye end of a sewing needle or similar metal object. Hold the needle with pliers, and use a match or lighter to heat it until the metal is red-hot. Press the glowing end of the needle against the nail so that it melts through. Little pressure is needed. The nail has no nerves, so this treatment is painless. **Figure 8**

(continued)

What to Look for	What to Do
	OR · Using a rotary action, carefully drill through the nail with the sharp point of a knife. This method may be painful and takes more time. 2. Apply a dressing to absorb the draining blood and to protect the injured nail.

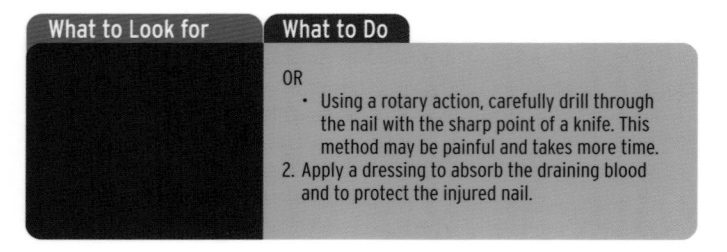

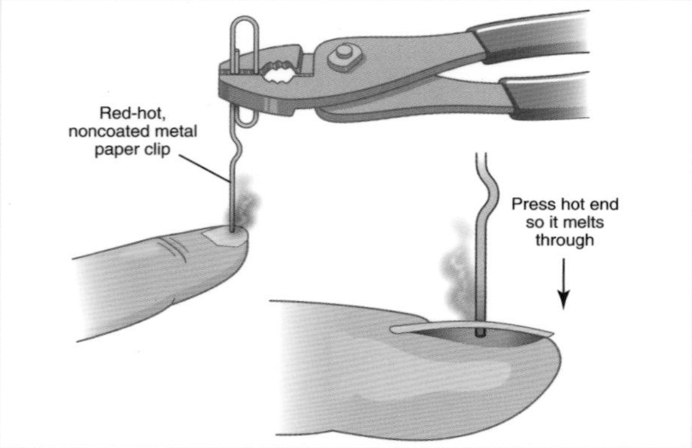

Red-hot, noncoated metal paper clip

Press hot end so it melts through

Figure 8

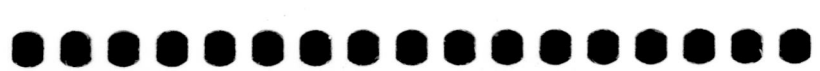

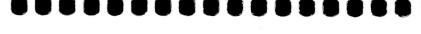

Amputations

What to Look for	What to Do

If a body part is amputated, immediate action is needed for reattachment. Amputated body parts that are left uncooled for more than 6 hours have little chance of survival.	1. Control the bleeding. Treat for shock by laying the victim down and keeping him/her covered.
	2. Recover the amputated part, and take it with the victim.
	3. Care for the amputated part:
	  • If possible, rinse part with clean water; **DO NOT** scrub.
	  • Wrap part with a moistened (not soaked) sterile gauze or clean cloth.
	  • Put the wrapped, amputated part in a plastic bag or another waterproof container.
	  • Place bag or container with the wrapped part in a container with ice. **DO NOT** bury the part in ice or allow it to directly touch the ice. **DO NOT** submerge it in water.
	4. Seek medical help ASAP.

Animal Bites

Use the procedures found in the *Bleeding and Wound Care* section. Animal bites have a high risk for infection; seek medical help.

Blisters

The following procedures are for friction blisters; **DO NOT** use for blisters related to poison ivy, burns, or frostbite.

What to Look for	What to Do
"Hot" spot (red, painful area caused by rubbing before blister formation)	Depending upon availability and the blister's location, use any of these products: • **Micropore paper tape:** Paper tape can be applied over and around toes and heels, sides, and backs of feet. Only paper tape should be used on toe blisters. It can be used underneath thicker tape. It is inexpensive, easy to use, and has a silky feel, but is not well suited for wet environments. • **Spenco 2nd Skin:** This is a gel pad. Follow the package's directions, which say to remove the cellophane from the side of the pad to be applied to the affected area and secure with the adhesive knit bandage found in the package or Elastikon. • **Moleskin and molefoam:** Moleskin has heavy cotton fabric on one side and adhesive backing on the other. Molefoam has foam material on one side and adhesive backing on the other. While they are commonly found in first aid kits, using these products has been criticized. Cut a hole in the middle of a pad the size of the "hot" spot and trim the corners to create a doughnut shape pad. Place the hole over the "hot" spot. Secure with tape. Some recommend stacking two layers of moleskin or molefoam to increase the thickness. The intent is to keep pressure off of the "hot" spot. • **Elastikon:** This is flexible tape made of a porous, cotton elastic cloth tape with a rubber-based adhesive. It is useful over heels and soles of feet. • **Duct tape:** This is strong and easy to apply. It is useful on the heel. It is not very breathable, which

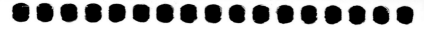

What to Look for	What to Do
	affects the skin underneath. It wrinkles easily and is difficult to remove. **DO NOT** use adhesive strips (i.e., Band-Aid) because they allow rubbing or friction between the skin and the nonadherent pad.
Blister on foot is closed and not very painful (collection of fluid in a "bubble" under outer layer of skin caused by rubbing)	Depending upon availability and the blister's location, use the most appropriate method described above.
Blister on the foot is open or is a very painful closed blister affecting the ability to walk	**For a very painful, closed blister:** 1. Clean area with soap and water or alcohol pad. 2. Clean a needle or knife with an alcohol pad or a match flame (let the blade cool before using). 3. Drain all of the fluid by making several small holes at base of blister with the needle or knife point. Press the fluid out. **DO NOT** remove the blister's roof unless it is torn. Apply an antibiotic ointment and cover the area with a sterile dressing. **For an open or torn blister:** 1. If torn, use scissors to carefully cut the blister roof's dead skin (it is not sensitive to pain). Place a piece of Spenco 2nd Skin over the area and cover with the adhesive knit bandage found in the package or Elastikon. If Spenco 2nd Skin is not available, apply antibiotic ointment and cover the area with a sterile dressing.

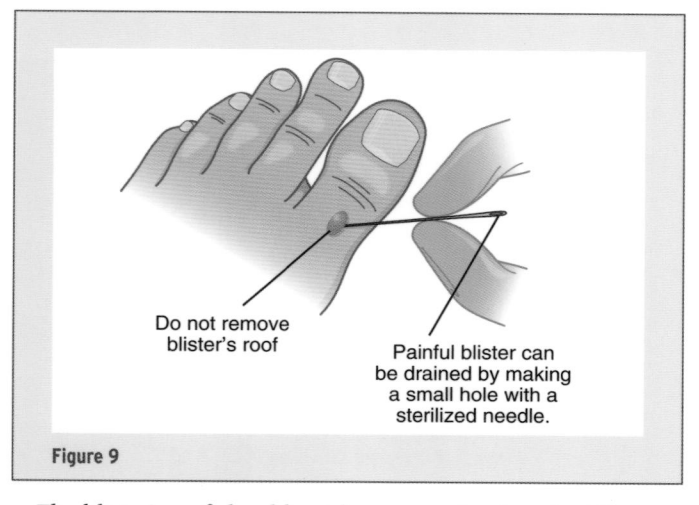

Do not remove
blister's roof

Painful blister can
be drained by making
a small hole with a
sterilized needle.

Figure 9

The blister's roof should not be removed unless the blister
is infected or is partially torn off. In these instances, use
sterilized scissors to remove the loose skin of the blister's
roof up to the edge of the normal skin, and apply antibiotic
ointment and a sterile dressing.

Fishhook Removal

DO NOT try to remove a fishhook if it is near an eye, if the
victim is uncooperative, or if you suspect that it is near a
major blood vessel or nerve. Warning signs include pulsating

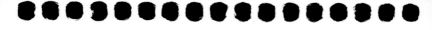

movement of the hook or numbness and tingling. If the barb has not penetrated the skin, back the hook out, and treat the wound. If the hook's barb has entered the skin, use one of these methods:

1. Seek medical help if it is nearby, and have a physician remove it.
2. If you are in a remote area more than 1 hour away from medical help, remove the hook using either the pliers method or the fish line method. After removing the hook, clean the wound and seek medical help. **Figure 10**

Internal Bleeding

Internal bleeding is difficult to recognize. The victim may have received a hard blow or penetrating object to the chest or abdomen.

What to Look for	What to Do
Pale, cool skin Affected area may be discolored, tender, and swollen. Fast breathing and heart rate Nausea and vomiting Blood may be seen as: · Red and foaming during coughing · Red or brown during vomiting · Black and tarry during bowel movement · Red or smoky brown during urinating · Oozing from the nose or ear · A black eye(s)	1. Monitor the vital signs (i.e., breathing and heart rates). 2. Treat for shock—elevate legs and maintain body heat. 3. If unresponsive or vomiting, place on side. 4. Seek medical help ASAP. **DO NOT** give food or drink.

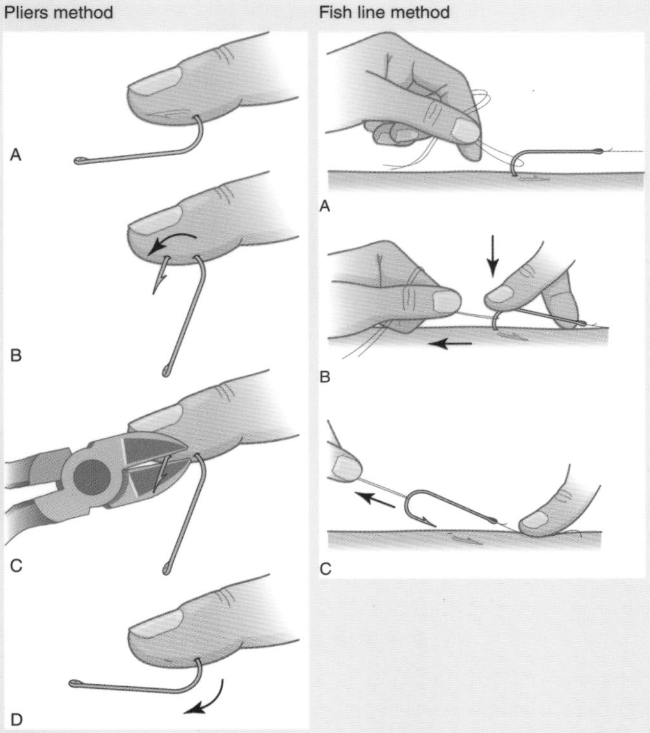

Pliers method

A

B

C

D

Fish line method

A

B

C

Figure 10

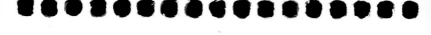

■ Bone, Joint, and Muscle Injuries

Broken Bones (Fractures)

RICE Procedures

Use RICE for bone, joint, and muscle injuries. In addition to RICE, fractures and dislocations should be stabilized against movement with a splint. **Figures 11 and 12**

R = Rest. The victim should not use the injured part.

I = Ice. Cold should be applied as soon as possible for 20 to 30 minutes every 2 to 3 hours during the first 24 to 48 hours. Cold sources include ice and cold water. Put a thin cloth or paper towel between the ice and skin to protect the skin from excessive cold.

C = Compression. Applying an elastic bandage reduces swelling. When not applying cold, apply compression (pressure). Place soft padding around the bones to compress the soft tissues to help reduce swelling.

E = Elevation. If possible, keep the injured part higher than the heart to reduce swelling and pain.

What to Look for	What to Do
It may be difficult to tell whether a bone is broken. When in doubt, treat the injury as a broken bone. Use "DOTS" to check an injury:	1. Gently remove any clothing covering injured area.
	2. Check blood flow and nerves—for arm, feel for heartbeat at the wrist; for leg, feel for heartbeat behind inside ankle knob. Ask the victim whether he or she feels you lightly

(continued)

What to Look for

- **D**eformity might be obvious. Compare the injured part with the uninjured part on the other side.
- **O**pen wound may have an underlying broken bone.
- **T**enderness and pain will be easily pointed out by the victim. A useful technique for detecting a fracture is to gently feel, touch, or press along the length of the bone; a victim's report of tenderness or pain can indicate a fracture.
- **S**welling happens rapidly after a fracture.

What to Do

squeezing the toes/fingers; ask the victim to wiggle the toes/fingers unless injured.
3. Use RICE procedures (discussed on the next page).
4. Give pain medication.
5. If there is mild or no significant deformity, stabilize in place by applying a splint.
6. If there is a significant deformity, gently realign the limb and then splint.
7. Seek medical help if victim cannot continue trip.

Seek medical help ASAP for:
- Open fractures (bleeding)
- No arm/leg pulse
- Broken thigh (femur) or pelvic bone

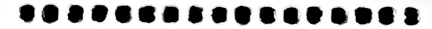

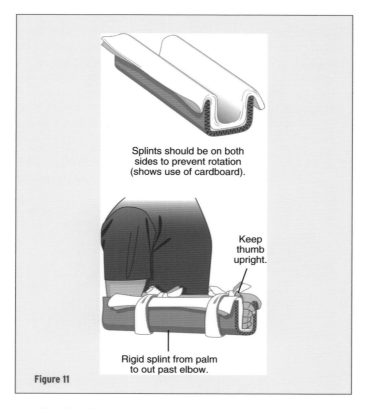

Splints should be on both
sides to prevent rotation
(shows use of cardboard).

Keep
thumb
upright.

Rigid splint from palm
to out past elbow.

Figure 11

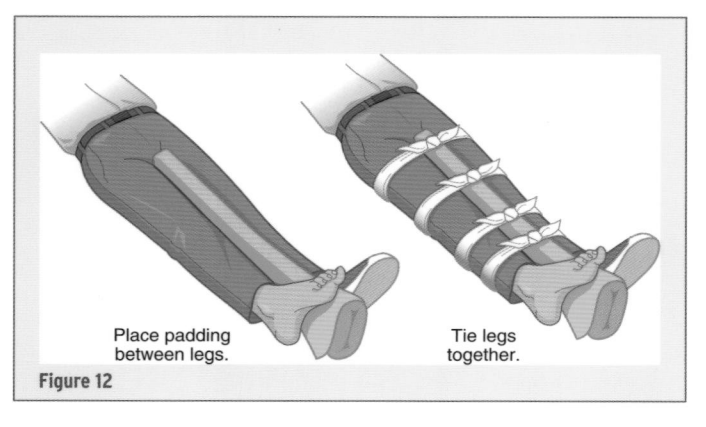

Place padding between legs.

Tie legs together.

Figure 12

Dislocated Joints: Shoulder, Kneecap, and Finger

A dislocation happens when a joint (e.g., shoulder, finger) comes apart and stays apart. Joint deformity is usually obvious. Relocation should only be attempted for dislocated shoulders, kneecaps (not to be confused with knee joints), and fingers. Relocate as soon as possible because it is easier before swelling and muscle spasms develop. **DO NOT** try to relocate elbows, hips, ankles, wrists, or knees. It is difficult to distinguish a dislocation from a severe fracture, and methods are painful and likely to cause further injury.

What to Look for	What to Do

Anterior shoulder (95% of all shoulder dislocations)
• Victim cannot touch opposite shoulder with hand of injured arm
• Arm held away from body
• Extreme pain
	1. Check heart rate at the wrist. Ask the victim whether he/she feels you lightly squeezing fingers; ask the victim to wiggle the fingers unless injured.
	2. Use one of the following methods:
	  • Simple hanging with 5 to 10 pounds of weight strapped to the wrist and lower arm (takes up to 60 minutes to work) **Figure 13**
	  OR
	  • Traction and rotation. Slowly move arm into a "baseball throwing" position above the head (takes up to 10 minutes). **Figure 14**
	3. After reduction, stabilize shoulder with arm sling.

Patella (kneecap) • The kneecap moved to the outside of knee joint (large bulge visible under skin) • Extreme pain	1. Bend hip toward chest and straighten leg. 2. You may need to push the kneecap back in place while straightening leg. 3. Splint with leg straight. The victim can usually walk on an injured leg.
Finger • Deformity (compare with the finger on the victim's opposite hand) • Inability to use	1. Hold the end of the finger, and pull it in the direction it is pointing. **Figure 15** 2. While pulling, swing the finger back into normal alignment. You may have to hyperextend the joint first. 3. Splint with "buddy taping" with fingers slightly bent and gauze between them. **Figure 16** Note: • Try reducing only once. • **DO NOT** try reducing joint at base of index finger or base of thumb (both require surgery).

Seek medical help for any shoulder, finger, or kneecap dislocations that cannot be relocated, and any dislocations of the wrist, elbow, hip, knee, and ankle.

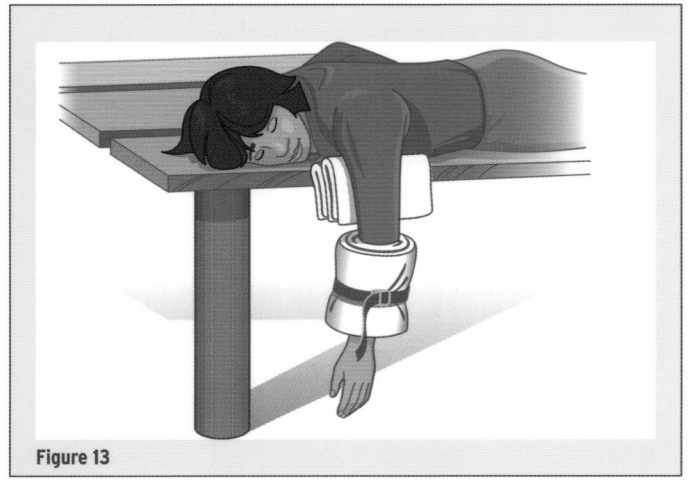

Figure 13

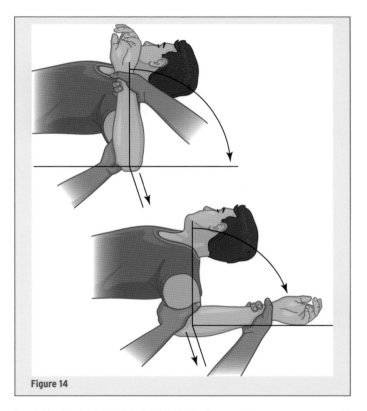

Figure 14

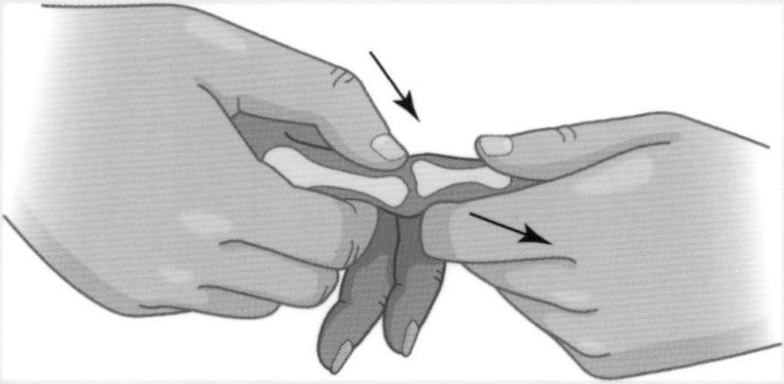

Figure 15

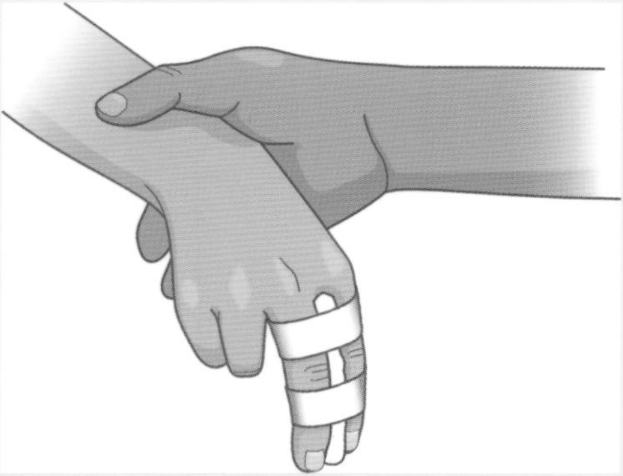

Figure 16
Modified from D.A. Auerbach, **Medicine for the Outdoors, Second Edition**, Little, Brown and Company.

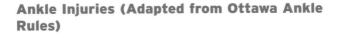

Ankle Injuries (Adapted from Ottawa Ankle Rules)

What to Look for	What to Do
Any pain or tenderness in ankle and 1. Bone tenderness along the back edge or tip of the ankle knob bone (malleolus), and 2. Cannot bear weight and take four steps immediately after the injury or an hour later.	Suspect fractured ankle 1. Treat with RICE. 2. Stabilize against movement with a splint. 3. Seek medical help.
Any pain or tenderness in ankle and 1. No bone tenderness along back edge or tip of ankle knob bone (malleolus) and 2. Can bear weight and take four steps immediately after the injury and an hour later.	Suspect sprained ankle 1. Treat with RICE. 2. No evacuation is usually needed. 3. **DO NOT** apply heat until 48 to 72 hours after injury. Figure 17

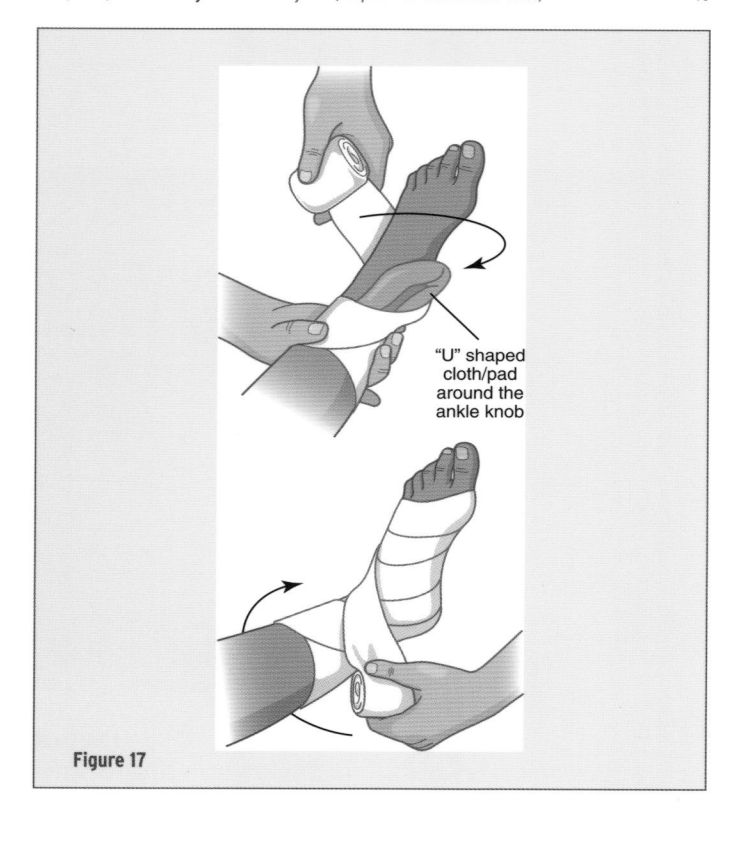

"U" shaped cloth/pad around the ankle knob

Figure 17

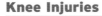

Knee Injuries

What to Look for	What to Do
Use one of these procedures to check for a knee injury: 1. Pittsburgh Knee Rules If a blunt trauma or a fall caused the injury, plus one of the following: · Age < 12 years or > 50 years · Inability to walk four steps 2. Ottawa Knee Rules: · Age > 55 years · Tenderness at the patella (kneecap) · Tenderness at head of fibula (bony knob on outside of knee · Inability to flex knee to 90 degrees · Inability to bear weight and take four steps immediately after injury or an hour later	3. Treat with RICE. 4. Stabilize against movement with splint. 5. Seek medical help.

Splinting Guidelines

All broken bones and dislocations should be stabilized before moving the victim. When in doubt, apply a splint. Any device can be used to stabilize a broken bone or dislocation. The device can be improvised (e.g., ski poles, canoe/kayak paddles,

or pillow) or can be a commercial splint (e.g., a SAM Splint).
A self-splint is one in which the injured body part is tied to an
uninjured part (e.g., injured finger taped to adjacent finger,
legs tied together, or arm tied to chest).

1. Cover open wounds with a dry, sterile dressing.
2. Check blood flow and nerves—for an arm, feel for a
   heartbeat at the wrist; for a leg, feel for a heartbeat behind
   the ankle knob on the inside. Ask the victim whether he
   or she feels you lightly squeezing toes/fingers, and ask the
   victim to wiggle his or her toes/fingers unless injured.
3. Determine what to splint by using the "Rule of Thirds."
   Imagine each long bone as being divided into thirds.
   If the injury is located in the upper or lower third of a
   bone, assume that the nearest joint is injured. Therefore,
   the splint should extend to stabilize the bones above and
   below the joint. For a break of the middle third of a bone,
   stabilize the joints above and below the fracture. A broken
   arm, in addition to being splinted, should be placed in an
   arm sling and binder (ties arm to chest).
4. If two first aid providers are present, one should
   support the injured part to minimize movement until
   splinting is finished.
5. If possible, place splint materials on both sides of the
   injured part, especially when two bones are involved (e.g.,
   radius and ulna, tibia and fibula) to prevent bone rotation.

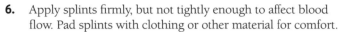

6. Apply splints firmly, but not tightly enough to affect blood flow. Pad splints with clothing or other material for comfort.

7. Try to straighten a fracture only in remote locations and if one or both of the following exists: (1) an extremity is badly deformed and/or (2) no heartbeat can be felt in the injured extremity. **DO NOT** move a suspected injured spine or replace a dislocation, *except* anterior shoulder, kneecap, and finger dislocations.

Muscle Injuries

What to Look for	What to Do
• Sudden muscle pain • A muscle, often the calf muscle, that feels hard because of the muscle contraction • Often residual discomfort for a few hours	Suspect a muscle cramp (spasm). Try one or more of these to relax the muscle: 1. Have the victim gently stretch the affected muscle. 2. Press on the muscle. 3. Apply cold to the muscle. 4. For a calf muscle cramp only, have the victim pinch the upper lip hard (an acupressure technique). 5. Drink lightly salted cool water (one-fourth teaspoon salt in 1 quart of water) or commercial sports drinks.
• A blow to a muscle • Swelling • Tender and painful • Black and blue mark appears hours later	Suspect a muscle bruise (contusion). Use the RICE procedures. *(continued)*

What to Look for	What to Do
• Occurs during physical activity • Sharp pain • Very tender • Cannot use injured part • Stiffness and pain when muscle is used	Suspect muscle strain (pull). Use the RICE procedures.

Seek medical help for these injuries ASAP (adapted from the Wilderness Medical Society guidelines):

- A broken bone or dislocation with an open fracture
- No heartbeat felt in the extremity
- Suspected spinal cord injury
- Heavy blood loss
- Severe deformity affecting blood flow and/or sensation

Burns

1. Stop the burning! If clothing is on fire, have victim roll on the ground using the "stop, drop, and roll" method. Smother the flames with a blanket, or douse the victim with water. Remove clothing and all jewelry, especially rings, from the burn area. If it is a chemical burn, wash

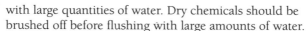

with large quantities of water. Dry chemicals should be brushed off before flushing with large amounts of water.

2. Check and monitor breathing if the victim breathed heated air or was in an explosion.
3. Determine the depth of the burn. This is difficult but helps determine what first aid to give.
4. Determine the size of the burn by using the "Rule of the Hand." The victim's hand (includes palm, closed fingers, and thumb) equals about 1% of victim's body surface area (BSA).
5. Determine which parts of the body are burned. Burns on the face, hands, feet, and genitals are more severe than burns on other body parts.

What to Look for	What to Do
First-degree burn (superficial) • Redness • Mild swelling • Tenderness • Pain	1. Immerse the burned area in cold water, or apply a wet, cold cloth until pain-free both in and out of the water. If cold water is unavailable, use any cold liquid available. 2. Give ibuprofen (for children, give acetaminophen). 3. Have the victim drink as much water as possible without becoming nauseous. 4. Keep burned arm or leg raised. 5. After burn has been cooled, apply aloe vera gel or an inexpensive moisturizer. First-degree burns do not need to be covered.

(continued)

What to Look for	What to Do
Small second-degree burn of less than 20% BSA (partial-thickness) • Blisters • Swelling • Weeping of fluids • Severe pain	1. Follow same procedures (steps 1 through 4) as for a first-degree burn, with these additions: 2. After burn has been cooled, apply thin layer of antibacterial ointment (e.g., Bacitracin or Neosporin). 3. Cover burn with a dry, nonsticking, sterile dressing or a clean cloth.
Large second-degree burn or more than 20% BSA (partial-thickness burn)	1. Follow steps 2 through 4 of first-degree burn care. **DO NOT** apply cold because it may cause hypothermia. 2. Seek medical help.
Third-degree burn (full-thickness) • Dry, leathery, grayish, or charred skin	1. Cover burn with a dry, nonsticking, sterile dressing or clean cloth. 2. Seek medical help.

Evacuation

Most burns are minor and do not require medical help. Superficial and small partial-thickness burns rarely need medical help. Large partial-thickness and all full-thickness burns, burned airways, and circumferential burns (completely around body part) need medical help ASAP.

C

◼ Cardiac Arrest (Heart Stops)

CPR (Cardiopulmonary Resuscitation)

For a motionless person, use the mnemonic **RAB-CAB** to remember what to do. Start as soon as possible!

RAB

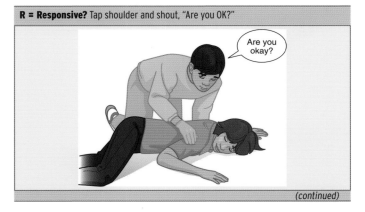

R = Responsive? Tap shoulder and shout, "Are you OK?"

Are you okay?

(continued)

If...	Then...
Unresponsive and only gasping or not breathing	CPR is needed. Go to step **A = Activate.**
Unresponsive and breathing normally	Place victim on his/her side and monitor breathing.

A = Activate EMS by asking another person(s) to go or call for help by using a cell phone, satellite phone, or radio. A whistle can attract nearby people's attention who might be able to help.

If...	Then...
Alone	**For adult:** Immediately try calling for help and get AED, if available. Then, return to victim to attach and use AED. **For child or infant:** Call after 5 cycles (2 minutes) of CPR.
Bystander or another rescuer is available	Send him/her to call or get help and AED, if available.

B = Breathing? Check for no breathing or only gasping. Observe person's chest for movement (rise and fall) for 5–10 seconds.

CAB

C = Chest compressions. Push hard and fast.

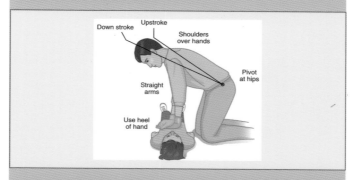

Where to place hands?
For adult: Use 2 hands. Place heel of one hand on breastbone in center of chest with other hand on top and interlock fingers.

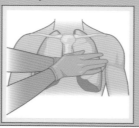

(continued)

For child: Use 1 or both hands in same place as for an adult.

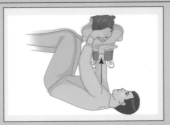

For infant: Place 2 fingers in the center of chest below nipple line, with one finger touching it.

How deep?
Push hard!
For adult: Push down on chest at least 2 inches (5 cm) to 2.4 inches (6 cm).
For child: About 2 inches (5 cm).
For infant: About 1.5 inches (3.8 cm).

Allow chest to come back up to its normal position after each compression.

How fast?
Push fast!
Push chest at same beat of the Bee Gee's song, "Stayin' Alive." Count at fast rate: "1, 2, 3, 4...30." This is at the rate of 100–120 compressions per minute.

How many?
Give 30 compressions without interruption unless AED arrives. If AED becomes available, use immediately.

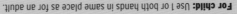

(continued)

A = Airway open. Open airway by tilting head back and lifting chin.

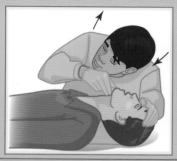

B = Breaths. Give 2 normal breaths (1 second each) that make chest rise.
For adult and child: Pinch victim's nose shut and make airtight mouth-to-mouth seal. Use CPR mask if available.

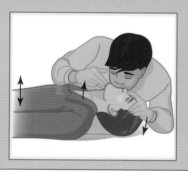

For infant: Cover mouth and nose with your mouth. If this does not work, try either mouth-to-mouth or mouth-to-nose.

If...	Then...
2 breaths make chest rise	Continue CPR: • 30 chest compressions (push hard and fast). • 2 breaths (1 second each). Take a regular breath, not a deep breath, between the 2 breaths. • Continue 30:2 compression to breath ratio until AED arrives and is ready to use, or until trained person takes over. • **DO NOT** stop to check for breathing until after 5 cycles of compressions and breaths.
First breath does not make chest rise; the airway may be blocked.	Retilt head, give a second breath • If second breath does not make chest rise, continue CPR. Each time the airway is opened to give a breath, look for an object in the victim's mouth and, if found, remove it.

Continue CPR until
- Victim begins breathing
- Trained rescuer(s) take over
- AED arrives and is used
- You are physically exhausted and unable to continue
- Scene becomes unsafe

Defibrillation

- Use AED as soon as possible.
- Expose chest, turn on AED, and attach pads.
- Follow voice directions.

If...	Then...
If no shock advised	Resume CPR immediately (evaluate again by AED after 5 sets of 30 compressions and 2 breaths).
If shock advised	**DO NOT** touch victim. Give 1 shock or shocks advised by AED. Resume CPR immediately starting with compressions.

Hands-Only (Compression-Only) CPR

What to Look for

If you see an adult or teen suddenly collapse and you are:
- Unable or unwilling to make mouth-to-mouth contact or
- Untrained in CPR.

What to Do

1. Check victim for gasping or no breathing.
2. Ask another person(s) to go or call for help.
3. Push center of chest hard and fast (faster than 1 per second).
4. Continue chest compressions until help arrives or as long as possible. If you get tired, switch with someone else (this may be every 2 minutes or 100 compressions).

CPR in Remote Locations

After cardiac arrest, a victim's heart activity must be restored within a short time (most require medical help) for survival; thus, CPR is seldom successful in remote locations. Nevertheless, you should start CPR when breathing stops.

If any of the following conditions* are present, **DO NOT** start CPR:
· The environment is unsafe and dangerous to rescuers
· Signs of death (e.g., rigor mortis or stiff, rigid muscles)
· Obvious lethal injury
· Documented do-not-resuscitate orders exist
· Victim has a rigid frozen chest
· Known time from incident to resuscitation is too long (30 minutes since heart stopped, more than 1 hour after submersion in water)

If ...	Then ...
CPR is started in a remote location*	Continue CPR until: · Victim recovers. · Rescuers are too exhausted to continue. · Another rescuer takes over. · Scene becomes unsafe and rescuers become endangered. · AED is ready to use. · A physician tells you to stop. · The victim does not respond to 30 minutes of resuscitation efforts (see below for exceptions).

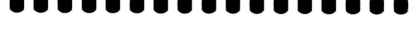

CPR is given for 30 minutes without success	Stop CPR. Exceptions when CPR should be given longer than 30 minutes: • Cold-water immersion of less than 1 hour • Avalanche burial • Hypothermia (for these victims, take 30 to 45 seconds to feel for a neck pulse before starting CPR) • Lightning strike

* Wilderness Medical Society guidelines

AED (Automated External Defibrillator)

Over 90% of cardiac arrest victims are in ventricular fibrillation (ineffective heart muscle contractions). Early defibrillation is the single most important factor in saving lives from sudden cardiac arrest. CPR alone will not reverse cardiac arrest, but it does buy time by allowing an AED to arrive and be applied. Most remote locations will not have an AED readily available due to its weight, bulk, and cost. In urban areas, using CPR and an AED can save lives, but in remote locations, this combination will usually not revive a victim unless there is fast access to a hospital—most victims will die. Because of these limitations, it is important to know when to start and stop giving CPR.

Give CPR until an AED arrives and is ready to use. Before using an AED, check for water or puddles around the victim. Most AEDs use the same steps for adults, children, and infants:

1. Turn on AED.
2. Attach the pads (as shown on the pads) on the victim's bare, dry chest. If needed, plug the cables into the AED.
3. Stay clear of the victim. Make sure no one, including you, is touching the victim. Say, "Clear!"
4. Allow the AED to analyze the heart rhythm (push "analyze" button, if necessary).
5. AED prompts one of three actions: (a) press shock button, (b) stay clear while AED automatically delivers a shock, or (c) do not shock but give CPR starting with chest compressions with the pads staying in place.
6. After any one of the three actions, give 5 cycles of CPR (takes about 2 minutes when AED says to stop to analyze heart rhythm), unless the victim moves, begins to breathe, or wakes up.
7. Repeat steps 3 through 6 until the victim starts to move, wakes up, or begins to breathe, or if more highly trained rescuers take over.

■ Chest Injuries

Chest injuries can involve broken bones, penetrating injuries, and open or closed wounds.

For all chest injuries, look for the following:

• DOTS: deformity, open wounds, tenderness, and swelling.

- Abnormal breathing rate and/or sounds (i.e., gurgling).
- Guarding (protecting an area during moving or touching).

Rib Fractures

What to Look for	What to Do

- Sharp pain when victim takes deep breaths, coughs, or moves
- Victim holding area, trying to reduce pain
- Tenderness.
- Shallow breathing because normal or deep breathing hurts
- Bruising of skin over the injury
- Usually occurs along the side of the chest
	1. Help victim find a comfortable position.
	2. Stabilize chest by:
	   a. Having victim hold a pillow or other similarly soft material against the area, or
	   b. Placing arm on the injured side in a sling and binder (swathe) if necessary for pain control
	3. **DO NOT** apply tight bandages around the chest.
	4. Give pain medication.
	5. Have victim cough and take deep breaths, even if it hurts, a few times every hour to prevent pneumonia.
	6. Seek medical help.

Flail Chest

A flail chest happens when several ribs in the same area are broken in more than one place.

What to Look for	What to Do
- Area over the injury may move in a direction opposite to that of the rest of the chest wall during breathing.	1. Stabilize chest by: a. Placing a pillow or similarly soft material against area or arm on the injured side in a sling and binder (swathe) and *(continued)*

What to Look for	What to Do
· Very painful and difficult breathing · Bruising of skin over the injury · Same as for Rib Fractures	b. Placing the victim on his/her injured side with a blanket or similarly soft material underneath the victim. 2. **DO NOT** apply tight bandages around the chest. 3. Seek medical help.

Penetrating Object in Chest

What to Look for	What to Do
· Usually easy to see impaled object	1. Stabilize object in place with bulky dressings or clothes. **DO NOT** try to remove the object. 2. Seek medical help.

Open Chest Wound

What to Look for	What to Do
· Blood bubbling out of a chest wound during exhalation · Sucking sound heard during inhalations	1. Open chest wounds require immediate evacuation to a medical facility. 2. DO NOT apply a dressing to close off an open chest wound—leave the wound exposed to the air without a dressing or seal. 3. If a non-sealing dressing (i.e., dry gauze dressing) is applied for bleeding, avoid blood saturation of the dressing that leads to closing off the wound. 4. Lean or lay victim on the injured side.

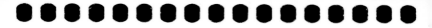

Chest Pain

What to Look for	What to Do
Muscle or rib pain from physical activity or injury	1. Have the victim rest. 2. Apply cold to the affected area. 3. Give pain medication.
Respiratory infection (bronchitis, pleuritis, pneumonia) · Cough · High fever and shaking chills, which are a sign of bacterial infection · Sore throat · Production of thick green or yellow sputum is a sign of bacterial infection.	1. Antibiotics are usually needed for bacterial infections and may be given if available. 2. Antibiotics are not needed for viral infections. 3. Give fluids and pain medications. 4. Seek medical care if the victim is worsening or having difficulty breathing.
Indigestion · Belching · Heartburn · Nausea · Sour taste	1. Give antacids.
Angina pectoris (chest pain lasting less than 10 minutes)	1. Have the victim rest. 2. Ask the victim if he/she takes any chest pain medication for a known heart condition, such as nitroglycerin, and help him/her take it. *(continued)*

What to Look for

Heart attack (see *Heart Attack* section)

- Chest pain in center of chest
- Sweating
- Light-headedness
- Nausea or vomiting
- Numbness, aching, or tingling in the arm
- Shortness of breath
- Weakness or fatigue

What to Do

1. Have the victim sit, with knees raised, and lean against a stable support (i.e., fence post, tree trunk). Try to keep the victim calm. **DO NOT** allow the victim to walk.
2. Loosen any tight clothing.
3. Ask if the victim takes any chest pain medication for a known heart condition, such as nitroglycerin, and help him/her take it.
4. If the victim is alert, able to swallow, and not allergic to aspirin, help the victim take one adult aspirin (325 mg) or four baby aspirins (81 mg each). Pulverize or have the victim crunch them with his/her teeth before swallowing for faster results.
5. Monitor breathing. If the victim becomes unresponsive and stops breathing, begin CPR (see *Cardiac Arrest* section for CPR).
6. Seek medical help ASAP.

■ Choking

1. Check victim for choking. Ask "Are you choking? Can you speak to me?" A choking victim may be clutching the neck with one or both hands (this is the universal choking sign). A choking victim cannot breathe, talk, cry, or cough.

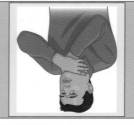

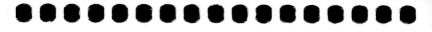

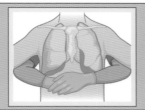

2. Give abdominal thrusts (Heimlich maneuver).
   - Stand behind victim and wrap your arms around the victim's waist. Give chest thrusts to a choking victim who is too big for you to reach around or who is pregnant.
   - Place a fist against the victim's abdomen, just above navel with your knuckles up.
   - Grasp your fist with your other hand and press your fist into victim's abdomen with quick inward and upward thrusts.
   - Continue thrusts until object is forced out or victim becomes unresponsive.

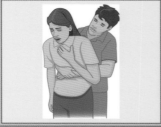

3. If victim becomes unresponsive and collapses onto ground:
   - Begin CPR.
   - After 30 compressions and each time you open the airway to give breaths, look for an object in the throat, and if seen, remove it.
4. For an infant who is choking, give chest thrusts in the same way you would for CPR chest compressions as described above.

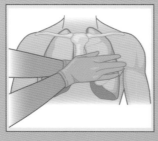

Leaves: © javarman/ShutterStock, Inc.

■ Diabetic Emergencies

When the body has too much sugar (glucose) present in the blood, the person is said to have diabetes mellitus, or simply "diabetes."

Before going into remote locations, a person with diabetes should tell the group's leader that he/she has diabetes; discuss the planned trip with his/her physician; and carry adequate supplies of necessary medicines and other equipment (i.e., insulin, syringes, needles, pills, etc.), including extra supplies for emergencies. An injectable medication called glucagon can raise blood sugar in an emergency. Another group member might agree to carry these extra supplies, and should be taught how to test blood sugar and inject glucagon in case the person with diabetes becomes incapacitated. Insulin and glucagon should be protected from the cold (in an inside pocket in cold weather) or heat (in a closed vacuum bottle or buried in the pack). A person with diabetes should also carry extra food and snacks, so that he/she does not have to rely on others in the group if food is needed quickly. **Figure 18**

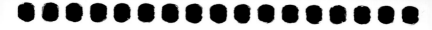

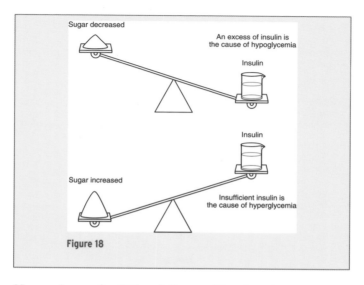

Figure 18

Hypoglycemia (Blood Sugar Too Low)

Hypoglycemia is a life-threatening emergency caused when the person with diabetes does any one of the following:

- Takes too much insulin (rapidly depletes sugar)
- Does not eat (reduces sugar intake)
- Overexerts him/herself or exercises (uses sugar faster)
- Vomits (empties stomach of sugar)

Most people with diabetes monitor their blood glucose levels as often as four times a day to maintain the proper levels and to prevent a diabetic emergency. Hypoglycemia can rapidly progress to a life-threatening situation.

What to Look for

- Medical identification tag
- Sudden onset (minutes to an hour) because no sugar is reaching the brain
- Staggering, poor coordination, clumsiness
- Anger, bad temper
- Cold, pale, moist, or "clammy" skin
- Confusion, disorientation
- Sudden hunger
- Excessive sweating
- Trembling, shakiness
- Seizure (no sugar reaching the brain)
- Eventual unresponsiveness

What to Do

If the person is responsive, alert, and can swallow:

1. The person may be able to tell you what to do. His/her blood sugar should be checked. If it is low, use the "rule of 15s" by having the person eat 15 grams of sugar (i.e., 3 to 5 glucose tablets, 3 to 5 tsp. of table sugar, 1 tube of glucose gel, 2 tbsp. of raisins, or 4 oz. of orange or apple juice). If the person with diabetes is not able to test his/her blood glucose, and you strongly suspect that the person has low blood glucose, give him/her 15 grams of fast-acting sugar.

2. Wait 15 minutes for the sugar to get into the blood.

3. The blood glucose level should be rechecked. If it is still low, he/she should consume 15 more grams of sugar. If testing is not available, and there is no improvement in 15 minutes after the first 15 grams of sugar, give 15 more grams of sugar.

(continued)

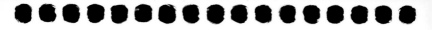

What to Look for	What to Do
	4. If there is no improvement, seek medical help ASAP.
	If the person is unresponsive:
	1. Place the person onto his or her side.
	2. If available, give glucagon.
	3. Place glucose gel or a paste made of water and sugar between a cheek and the gum, where it may be swallowed reflexively, or rub sugar into the his/her gums where some may be absorbed into the blood. These procedures may take some time to start working, so do not give up too quickly.
	4. If there is no improvement, seek medical help ASAP.

Hyperglycemia (Blood Sugar Too High)

This condition occurs when a person with diabetes has too much sugar in their blood. Several conditions can cause this (i.e., insufficient insulin, overeating, illness, inactivity, stress, or a combination of these factors). Hyperglycemia in remote locations is rarely encountered unless a person with diabetes is stranded and has either lost or run out of his/her diabetes medication. Hyperglycemia can be fatal if it is not treated within 24 hours.

What to Look for	What to Do
• Medical identification tag • Gradual onset (hours to days) because some sugar is still reaching the brain • Drowsiness • Extreme thirst • Very frequent urination • Warm, red, dry skin • Vomiting • Fruity breath odor (has also been described to be like nail polish remover) • Heavy breathing • Eventual unresponsiveness	Most people with diabetes can recognize what is happening and will adjust their insulin dose or seek medical help before serious problems develop. 1. Give frequent, small sips of water if the person with diabetes can swallow. 2. If uncertain whether the person with diabetes has a high or low blood sugar level, and he/she is responsive and able to swallow, use the "rule of 15s" for giving sugar described previously. "Sugar (glucose) for everyone" is the rule of thumb for all diabetic emergencies–hyper- or hypoglycemia. You do not need to distinguish between them. The extra sugar will not cause any significant harm in the person experiencing hyperglycemia. 3. **DO NOT** give insulin unless the person with diabetes can self-administer it. 4. Seek medical help ASAP.

Drowning (Submersion/Immersion)

Hypothermic victims submerged less than 60 minutes may respond to prolonged resuscitation, but generally only if they can be rewarmed, which may be impractical in the wilderness. If medical help is available rapidly, CPR should be continued

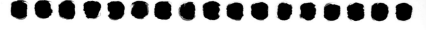

until the victim has been rewarmed. In hypothermic victims submerged more than 60 minutes, CPR is rarely successful.

What to Look for	What to Do
• Person floating on surface of water and waving for help • A struggling swimmer who suddenly becomes motionless in the water • A person who dives under the water and never reappears	1. Rescue by using "reach, throw, row, go." • Reach = Reach with a long object (e.g., tree limb or paddle) from shore. • Throw = Throw any object that floats (e.g., picnic jug or spare tire) or throw a rope and tow the victim to safety. • Row = Use a rowboat, raft, or canoe if available. • Go = If trained and skilled, swim to the victim. Use a towel or board for him or her to hold onto. **DO NOT** let the victim grab you. This can be a dangerous rescue. 2. Check for breathing, and if not breathing, perform CPR. 3. Check for spinal cord injury for the victim who dove into water; protect the spine if a spinal injury is suspected (see the *Spinal Injury* section). 4. Seek medical help ASAP even if victim feels "okay." 5. Stop CPR after 30 minutes unless the victim is hypothermic and has been submerged for less than 60 minutes.

Leaves: © javarman/ShutterStock, Inc.

■ Ear Injuries

Objects Stuck in an Ear

Except for disc batteries and live insects, few foreign bodies must be removed immediately. **DO NOT** use tweezers or try to pry an object out. Seek medical help to remove an object. For a live insect in the ear canal, shine a small light into the ear. Sometimes the insect will crawl out toward the light. If it will not leave the ear, pour warm water into the ear and then drain it. This may drown the insect, but whether it is dead or alive, it should wash out. When draining the water, turn the head to the side. If an insect cannot be removed, seek medical help.

Fluids Coming From an Ear

Blood or clear fluid draining from an ear may indicate a skull fracture. **DO NOT** attempt to stop bleeding or clear fluid (known as cerebrospinal fluid [CSF]) with or without blood coming from an ear. Blocking blood or CSF could increase pressure on the brain, causing permanent damage. Place a sterile gauze dressing over the ear and loosely bandage it in place to prevent bacteria getting into the brain. Stabilize the head and neck against movement. Seek medical help ASAP.

■ Eye Injuries

DO NOT assume that an eye injury is minor. For double vision, pain, or reduced vision, seek medical help. When in doubt, seek medical help ASAP.

What to Look for	What to Do
Blow to eye	1. Keep the victim on his or her back with the eyes closed. 2. Apply cold around eye for 15 minutes.
Loose object in eye	1. Try, in order, each step until one is effective: • Pull the upper eyelid down and over the lower lid. • Pull lower lid down, and look at inner surface while victim looks up. If object is seen, remove it with wet gauze. • Lift the upper eyelid up and over a cotton swab (Q-tip). If an object is seen, remove it with wet gauze. • Gently irrigate with clean, warm water. 2. If successful, medical help is usually not needed. <div align="right">*(continued)*</div>

What to Look for	What to Do
Object stuck in eye	1. **DO NOT** remove the object. 2. If the object is long, place padding around object to stabilize against movement and place paper cup or similar object over eye for protection. If the object is short, place a doughnut-shaped pad around the eye and hold it in place with bandage wrapped around head. 3. To reduce movement of the injured eye, cover the uninjured eye with a bandage, but it may be necessary to leave a peephole to prevent anxiety. 4. Keep the victim flat on his or her back. 5. Seek medical help ASAP.
Eyeball cut	1. **DO NOT** apply pressure to eye. 2. Cover both eyes with gauze pads held by a bandage lightly wrapped around head. 3. Keep the victim's head raised. 4. Seek medical help ASAP.
Chemical, smoke, or other irritant in eye	1. Hold the eye wide open; flush with warm water for 20 minutes. 2. The eye(s) may need to be loosely bandaged. 3. Seek medical help ASAP for chemical injury.
Burns caused by light (from looking at sunlight or reflection off of snow or water); these burns may not be painful at first but become very painful hours later.	1. Cover both eyes with moist, cool cloths. 2. Give pain medication if needed. 3. Seek medical advice.

Leaves: © javarman/ShutterStock, Inc.

Female Health Problems

Vaginitis

What to Look for	What to Do
· White or yellowish discharge · Pain when urinating · Vaginal soreness, burning, and/or itching	1. The victim should wash several times daily with clean water. 2. She should wear loose-fitting underwear and pants. 3. She should wipe from front to back after a bowel movement or after urinating. 4. Seek medical help if there is lower abdominal pain and a fever or if foul-smelling vaginal discharge exists.

Urinary Tract Infection

What to Look for	What to Do
· Frequent urge to urinate · Burning while urinating · Blood in the urine	1. Give fluids—water is best. Avoid caffeine and alcohol. 2. The victim should wear loose-fitting underwear and pants. <div align="right">(continued)</div>

What to Look for	What to Do
	3. She should wash the area daily.
	4. A hot bath may help relieve pain and itching.
	5. She should wipe from front to back after a bowel movement or after urinating.
	6. Seek medical help if symptoms last for 24 hours or if fever and chills occur.

Vaginal Bleeding

For injury-related soft-tissue injuries, use direct pressure to control bleeding. Apply cold to reduce swelling and pain. Apply a diaper-type bandage to hold dressings in place. Never place or pack dressings into the vagina. Seek medical help. Noninjury vaginal bleeding can result from various causes, but the care is the same. Have the woman place a sanitary pad over the vaginal opening, and seek medical help.

Pregnancy Problems

- The "big three" warning signs of a serious problem are bleeding, abdominal cramps, and weakness. Seek medical help ASAP.
- Morning sickness, swollen ankles, and urinary tract infections are not usually dangerous, but seek medical advice.

- If a pregnant woman is "spotting," have her lie down on her left side because this improves circulation. Spotting could signal the onset of a miscarriage.

■ Frostbite and Frostnip

Freezing limited to the skin surface is frostnip. Freezing that extends deeper through the skin and into the flesh is frostbite.

Frostbite

Frostbite happens only in below-freezing temperatures. It mainly affects the feet, hands, ears, and nose. The most severe consequences of frostbite occur when tissue dies (gangrene) and the affected part might have to be amputated. The longer the tissue stays frozen, the worse the injury. Check for hypothermia in any frostbitten victim.

What to Look for	What to Do
The severity and extent of frostbite are difficult to judge until hours after thawing. Before thawing, frostbite can be classified as superficial or deep. *Superficial frostbite* signs and symptoms include: • The skin is white, waxy, or grayish-yellow.	All frostbite injuries require the same first aid treatment. 1. Get the victim out of the cold and to a warm place. If possible, do not use a frozen extremity until medical help is reached. 2. Remove any wet clothing and constricting items, such as rings, that could impair blood circulation. *(continued)*

What to Look for

- The affected part feels very cold and numb. There might be tingling, stinging, or an aching sensation.
- The skin surface feels stiff or crusty and the underlying tissue feels soft when depressed gently and firmly.

Deep frostbite signs and symptoms:

- The affected part feels cold, hard, and solid and cannot be depressed–it feels like a piece of wood or frozen meat.
- The affected part has pale, waxy skin.
- A painfully cold part suddenly stops hurting.

After thawing, frostbite can be categorized by degrees, similar to the classification of burns.

- First-degree: The affected part is warm, swollen, and tender.
- Second-degree: blisters form minutes to hours after thawing and enlarge over several days.
- Third-degree: blisters are small and contain reddish

What to Do

3. **DO NOT** attempt to thaw the part if: (a) medical help is less than 2 hours away; (b) the affected area has thawed; (c) shelter, warm water, and a container are not available; or (d) there is a risk of refreezing.
4. Use the below wet, rapid rewarming method if: (a) medical help is more than 2 hours away; (b) there is no possibility of refreezing the affected area, or (c) shelter, warm water, and a container are available. While rapid rewarming is recommended, slow thawing may be unavoidable and should be allowed if it is the only method available.

Wet, rapid, rewarming method: Place the frostbitten part in warm (100° to 104°F) water. **DO NOT** use other heat sources (i.e., fire, space heater, oven). If you do not have a thermometer, you can put your hand into the water for 30 seconds to test that it is warm, but not hot enough to burn. Maintain water temperature by adding warm water as needed. Rewarming usually takes 20 to 40 minutes or until the part becomes soft and pliable to touch and takes on a red/purple appearance. Air dry the area–**DO NOT** rub. To help control the severe pain during rewarming, give the victim ibuprofen. For ear or facial injuries, it is best to apply warm, moist cloths, changing them frequently.

(continued)

What to Look for

blue or purplish fluid. The surrounding skin can be red or blue and might not blanch when pressure is applied.

What to Do

Cautions:
- **DO NOT** rub or massage the affected area.
- **DO NOT** apply ice or snow or cold water.
- **DO NOT** rewarm with stove, vehicle's tailpipe exhaust, or over a fire.
- **DO NOT** break blisters.
- **DO NOT** allow the victim to smoke or drink alcohol.
- **DO NOT** rewarm if there is any possibility of refreezing.
- **DO NOT** allow the thawed part to refreeze because it results in greater damage (i.e., gangrene).

5. After thawing:
- If the feet are affected, treat the victim as a stretcher case—the feet will be impossible to use after they are rewarmed unless only the toes are affected.
- Protect the affected area from contact with clothing and bedding.
- Place bulky, dry, clean gauze on the affected part and between the toes and the fingers to absorb moisture and keep them from sticking together.
- Slightly elevate the affected part above heart level to reduce pain and swelling.
- Apply aloe vera gel to promote skin healing.
- Give ibuprofen to limit pain and inflammation.

(continued)

What to Look for	What to Do
	6. Give fluids if the victim is alert, can swallow, and has no gastrointestinal problems.
	7. Seek medical help ASAP.

Frostnip

Frostnip is caused when water on the skin surface freezes. Frostnip should be taken seriously because it could be the first sign of impending frostbite.

What to Look for	What to Do
It is difficult to tell the difference between frostnip and frostbite. Signs of frostnip include: • Yellowish to gray-colored skin • Frost (ice crystals) on the skin • Tingling or numbness initially, which can become painful	1. Get the victim out of the cold and to a warm place. 2. Gently warm the affected area by placing it against a warm body part (i.e., have victim put bare hands under the armpits) or by applying a warm chemical heat pack covered by a cloth. For the nose, breathe with cupped hands over the nose. 3. **DO NOT** rub the area.

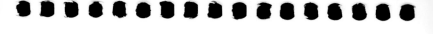

Immersion Foot

Immersion foot, also known as trench foot, occurs in nonfreezing cold and wet conditions. This takes several days to occur.

What to Look for	What to Do
Feet are: • Cold, swollen, pale • Numb • Blotched with dark splotches	1. Dry and warm feet. 2. Give fluids to drink. 3. Give ibuprofen. 4. Elevate the feet. 5. Seek medical help.

Leaves: © javarman/ShutterStock, Inc.

■ Head Injuries

Suspect a spinal cord injury in head injured victims. Stabilize against movement until you have "cleared" the spinal cord (see the section on *Spinal Injury*).

Scalp Wound

1. Control bleeding by pressing on wound. Replace any skin flap to its original position and apply pressure.
2. If you suspect a skull fracture, **DO NOT** apply excessive pressure; this may push bone pieces into the brain. Press on the edges of the wound to help control bleeding.
3. Apply a dry, sterile dressing.
4. Keep the head and shoulders raised if no spinal injury is suspected.
5. If medical help will be delayed and the wound is gaping open, twist small bundles of hair and tie them across the wound, drawing the edges snugly together.

6. If oozing continues, **DO NOT** remove the first blood-soaked dressing, but add another dressing over it.
7. Seek medical help if:

- The laceration is extensive.
- There is significant facial damage.
- Signs of a brain injury occur.

Skull Fracture

What to Look for	What to Do
· Pain · Skull deformity · Bleeding from an ear or the nose · Leakage of clear, watery fluid from an ear or the nose (CSF) · Discoloration around the eyes or behind ears appearing several hours after the injury · Unequal-sized pupils of the eye · Heavy scalp bleeding (skull and/or brain tissue may be exposed) · Penetrating or impaled object	If you suspect a skull fracture: 1. Monitor breathing. 2. Control bleeding by pressing the edges of the wound and gently on the center of it. 3. Cover wounds with a sterile dressing. 4. Stabilize the neck against movement unless you have "cleared" the spinal cord (see the section on *Spinal Injury*). 5. Seek medical help ASAP. *Cautions:* 　**DO NOT** clean the wound. 　**DO NOT** remove an embedded object. 　**DO NOT** stop blood or clear fluid that is draining from an ear or the nose. 　**DO NOT** press on the fractured area.

Brain Injury (Concussion)

A concussion is a type of traumatic brain injury (TBI) caused by a bump, blow, or jolt to the head that can change the way the brain normally works.

Most concussions (80% to 90%) resolve within 7 to 10 days, but some victims take much longer to recover.

What to Look for	What to Do

These may worsen over minutes or hours:
• Behavior or personality changes
• Blank stare/dazed look
• Changes to balance, coordination, reaction time
• Delayed or slowed spoken or physical responses
• Disorientation, memory loss (confused about date/location)
• Loss of responsiveness (occurs in fewer than 10% of concussions)
• Slurred/unclear speech
• Difficulty controlling emotions
• Vomiting
	1. If unresponsive, do a Primary Assessment (see *Finding Out What Is Wrong* section).
	2. If a neck injury exists or if the victim is unresponsive:
	  a. **DO NOT** move the head, neck, or spine.
	  b. Seek medical help.
	3. Seek medical help ASAP if the victim:
	  a. Looks very drowsy or cannot be awakened.
	  b. Has one pupil (the black part in the middle of the eye) that is larger than the other.
	  c. Has a seizure.
	  d. Cannot recognize people or places.
	  e. Becomes more and more confused, restless, or agitated.
	  f. Exhibits unusual behavior.
	  g. Becomes unresponsive (VPU on the AVPU scale).
	  h. Has a headache that gets worse and/or does not go away.
	(continued)

What to Look for	What to Do

The victim may report:
• Headache
• Fuzzy or blurry vision
• Nausea
• Dizziness
• Sensitivity to noise or light
	i. Has repeated vomiting or nausea.
	j. Has slurred speech.
	4. Following the injury, the victim should:
	  a. Get plenty of sleep at night and rest during the day.
	  b. Avoid visual and sensory stimuli, including video games and loud music.
	  c. Ease into normal activities slowly, not all at once.
	  d. Avoid strenuous physical activities that increase the heart rate or require a lot of concentration.
	  e. Avoid anything that could cause another blow to the head or body.
	  f. **DO NOT** use aspirin or anti-inflammatory medications such as ibuprofen or naproxen. due to the risk of bleeding. Acetaminophen (Tylenol) can be used for postconcussion headaches.

Heart Attack

In a heart attack, the heart muscle tissue dies because its blood supply has been severely reduced or stopped.

What to Look for

- Chest pain that feels like pressure, squeezing, or fullness, usually in the center of the chest. It may also be felt in the jaw, shoulder, arms, or back. It may last for more than a few minutes, or it may come and go.
- Sweating or "cold sweats"
- Light-headedness or dizziness
- Nausea or vomiting (more common in women)
- Numbness, aching, or tingling in the arm (usually the left arm)
- Shortness of breath
- Weakness or fatigue, especially in an older adult

Heart attacks are difficult to determine. One-third of all victims do not have chest pain.

Women are more likely than men to have shortness of breath, nausea and vomiting, and back or jaw pain.

What to Do

1. Have the victim sit, with knees raised, and lean against a stable support (i.e., fence post, tree trunk). Try to keep the victim calm. **DO NOT** allow the victim to walk.
2. Loosen any tight clothing.
3. Ask if the victim takes any chest pain medication, such as nitroglycerin, for a known heart condition, and help him/her take it.
4. If the victim is alert, able to swallow, and not allergic to aspirin, help the victim take one adult aspirin (325 mg) or four baby aspirins (81 mg each). Pulverize or have the victim crunch them with his/her teeth before swallowing for faster results.
5. Monitor breathing. If the victim becomes unresponsive and stops breathing, begin CPR (see *Cardiac Arrest* section for CPR).
6. Seek medical help ASAP.

■ Heat-Related Illnesses

Heat illnesses include a range of disorders. Some are common, but only heatstroke is life threatening. Untreated heatstroke results in death.

Heatstroke

Two Types of Heatstroke

There are two types of heatstroke: *classic* and *exertional.*

The common characteristics of *classic* heatstroke are as follows:

- Usually affects older people
- More common in those who are chronically ill or sedentary
- More likely in those who take certain prescription medications
- More likely in those who are abusing drugs or alcohol
- Common during heat waves
- The victims do not sweat.

The common characteristics of *exertional* heatstroke are as follows:

- Affects young, healthy individuals who are not acclimatized to the heat
- Usually occurs during strenuous activity
- Sweating is prevalent in about 50% of the victims.

What to Look for

- Extremely hot skin when touched—usually dry, but can be wet from sweating related to strenuous work or exercise.
- Altered mental status ranging from slight confusion, agitation, and disorientation to unresponsiveness.

What to Do

Heatstroke is life threatening and must be treated rapidly!

1. Move the victim from the hot environment to a cool, shaded area.
2. Remove clothing down to the victim's underwear.
3. Cool the victim quickly by any means possible. In some remote locations, prompt cooling might be difficult. Controversy exists about the best cooling method. In no way should cooling of the heatstroke victim be delayed if any of the below methods are possible.

Choose the most appropriate option:
   - Spray the victim with water and then fan. This method is not as effective in high-humidity conditions.
   - Apply cool, wet sheets or cloths.
   - Place cold packs against the large veins on the groin, armpits, and sides of the neck; this cools the body, regardless of humidity.
   - Immerse the victim's body in a stream, pond, or lake. Using this method or the next two methods can be dangerous because of a chance of drowning.
   - Place the victim in an ice bath; this cools the victim quickly, but it requires a great deal of ice—at least 80 pounds—to be effective. The need for a big enough tub also limits this method.

(continued)

What to Look for	What to Do
	• Placing the victim in a cool water bath (less than 60°F) can be successful if the water is stirred to prevent a warm layer from forming around the body. This is very effective in high-humidity conditions. 4. **DO NOT** give aspirin or acetaminophen, as they are ineffective in reducing the body temperature for heatstroke. 5. Stop cooling when mental status improves. 6. Monitor the victim frequently because high temperatures can rise again after cooling. 7. Seek medical help ASAP.

Heat Exhaustion

What to Look for	What to Do
• Sweating • Thirst • Fatigue • Flu-like symptoms (headache, body aches, and nausea) • Shortness of breath • Rapid heart rate It differs from heatstroke because the victim has (1) no altered mental status and (2) skin that is not hot, but clammy.	Suspect heat exhaustion: Uncontrolled heat exhaustion can evolve into heatstroke. 1. Move the victim to a cool, shaded area. 2. Have the victim remove excess clothing. 3. Have the victim drink cool fluids. 4. For more severe cases, give lightly salted cool water (dissolve one-fourth teaspoon salt in 1 quart of water) or commercial sports drink. **DO NOT** give salt tablets. *(continued)*

What to Look for	What to Do
	5. Cool the victim, but not as aggressively as for heatstroke.
	6. If no improvement is seen within 30 minutes, seek medical help. Recovery may take up to 24 hours.

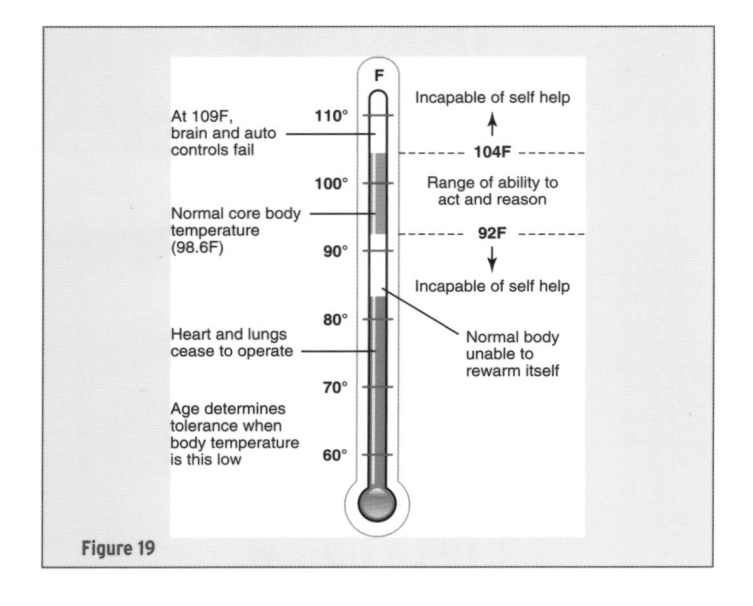

Figure 19

Hyponatremia ("Water Intoxication")

When sodium is flushed out of the body by drinking too much water, hyponatremia, nicknamed "water intoxication," can occur. Sodium loss is seldom a problem unless the victim sweats profusely for long periods and drinks large quantities of water.

What to Look for	What to Do
· The victim drank too much water (> 1 quart per hour) · Frequent urination; urine is clear · Profuse sweating for long periods · Dizziness, weakness, nausea, vomiting, headache · Altered mental status · Severe sodium loss may result in seizures or unresponsiveness, and can be fatal.	1. Move victim to a cool location. 2. **DO NOT** give more fluids unless you have added a pinch of salt in about 8 ounces of water. 3. Give salty foods. **DO NOT** give salt tablets because they can irritate the stomach and cause nausea and vomiting. 4. For altered mental status victims, seek medical help ASAP.

Heat Cramps

What to Look for

- Painful muscle spasms that happen suddenly
- Affects the muscle in the back of the leg or abdomen
- Occurs during or after physical exertion

What to Do

Relief may take several hours.
1. Have the victim rest in a cool area.
2. Drink lightly salted cool water (dissolve one-fourth teaspoon salt in 1 quart of water) or a commercial sports drink. **DO NOT** give salt tablets.
3. For any cramped muscle, stretch it. For calf muscles in the lower leg, stretch the cramped calf muscle and/or try the acupressure method of pinching the upper lip, just below the nose.

Heat Syncope

What to Look for

- Victim is dizzy or faints
- Occurs immediately after strenuous physical activity in a hot environment

What to Do

1. If the victim is unresponsive, check breathing. The victim usually recovers quickly.
2. If the victim fell, check for injuries.
3. Have the victim rest and lie down in a cool area.
4. Wet the skin by splashing water on the face.
5. If victim is not nauseated and if fully alert and able to swallow, give lightly salted cool water (dissolve one-fourth teaspoon salt in 1 quart of water) or a commercial sports drink. **DO NOT** give salt tablets.

Heat Edema

What to Look for	What to Do
· Swollen ankles and feet · Occurs during first few days in a hot environment.	1. Have victim wear support stockings. 2. Elevate victim's legs.

Heat Rash (Prickly Heat)

What to Look for	What to Do
· Itchy rash on skin wet from sweating · Seen in humid regions after prolonged sweating	1. Dry and cool victim's skin. 2. Limit heat exposure.

■ Hypothermia

Hypothermia happens when the body's temperature (98.6°F [37°C]) drops more than 2 degrees. Hypothermia does not require subfreezing temperatures. Severe hypothermia is life threatening. Check for possible frostbite.

Treat all hypothermic victims as follows:

1. Stop the heat loss:
   - Get the victim out of the cold.
   - Handle the victim gently.

- Replace wet clothing with dry clothing.
- Add insulation (e.g., blankets, towels, pillows, and sleeping bags) beneath and around the victim. Cover the victim's head.
- Cover the victim with a vapor barrier (e.g., tarp, plastic, and trash bags) to prevent heat loss. If unable to remove wet clothing, place a vapor barrier between clothing and insulation. For a dry victim, the vapor barrier can be placed outside of the insulation.

2. Keep the victim in a flat (horizontal) position.

Mild Hypothermia

What to Look for	What to Do
• Vigorous, uncontrollable shivering • The "umbles"—grumbles, mumbles, fumbles, stumbles • Cool or cold skin on abdomen, chest, or back	1. Follow steps 1 and 2 above for all hypothermic victims. 2. Allow the victim to shiver—**DO NOT** stop the shivering by adding heat. Shivering is desirable because it generates heat that will rewarm mildly hypothermic victims. 3. Give warm, sugary drinks, which can provide energy (calories) for the shivering to continue; they may also provide a psychologic boost. These drinks will not provide enough warmth to rewarm the victim. 4. **DO NOT** give alcohol to drink—it dilates blood vessels, allowing more heat loss. **DO NOT** allow tobacco use.

(continued)

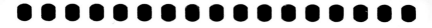

What to Look for	What to Do
	5. If the victim is adequately rewarmed and has a normal mental status, evacuation to medical help is usually not needed.

Severe Hypothermia

What to Look for	What to Do

· Rigid and stiff muscles
· No shivering
· Skin feels ice cold and appears blue
· Altered mental status
· Slow heart rate
· Slow breathing rate
· Victim may appear to be dead
	1. Follow steps 1 and 2 above for all hypothermic victims.
	2. Clothing on these victims should be cut off.
	3. Monitor breathing, and give CPR if necessary. Check the heart rate for 45 seconds before starting CPR.
	4. Very gently evacuate to medical help for rewarming. Rewarming in a remote location is difficult and rarely effective. However, when the victim is far from medical help, the victim must be warmed by any available external heat source (e.g., body-to-body contact).
	5. **DO NOT** start CPR if:
	  · The victim has been submerged in cold water for more than 1 hour
	  · This victim has obvious fatal injuries
	  · The victim is frozen (e.g., ice in airway)
	  · The victim has a chest that is stiff or that cannot be compressed
	  · Rescuers are exhausted or in danger

Additional cautions for hypothermic care are as follows:

1. **DO NOT** give a victim with altered mental status and decreased responsiveness any warm drinks because this may cause choking and inhalation of the liquid. If the victim is responsive enough to swallow, warm sugary drinks will help because they provide more calories to burn.
2. **DO NOT** rub the extremities.
3. **DO NOT** place the victim in a shower or bath.

Leaves: © javarman/ShutterStock, Inc.

Lightning Injuries

Lightning is an electrical discharge that is associated with thunderstorms. The "Rule of 70s" for lightning strikes indicates that 70% occur in the afternoons, 70% occur during the summer months, 70% survive but may be injured or burned, 70% have an aftereffect such as a hearing/visual/neurological impairment, and 70% involve only one victim.

Lightning kills by stopping the heart and breathing.

What to Look for	What to Do
• Lightning strike seen or thunder heard in area. Rain may or may not be present. • Minor burns on skin–the entrance and exit burn points common with electrical burns are rare with lightning. Types of burns:	Lightning victims are not "charged" and can be touched. 1. If more than one victim has been struck, first check the breathing of those who are not moving and quiet. 2. Give CPR to victims not breathing. 3. Check for spinal cord injury and treat. 4. If the victim is unresponsive but breathing, place him or her on his or her side. 5. Check for broken bones and dislocations and treat. *(continued)*

What to Look for

- Punctate: small circular injuries resembling cigarette burns-Feathering or ferning: looks like feather or fern leaf
- Linear burns
- Ignited clothing and heated-metal burns
• May appear confused
• Muscle aches and tingling
• May be unresponsive

What to Do

6. Check for burns and treat.
7. Seek medical help even if responsive.

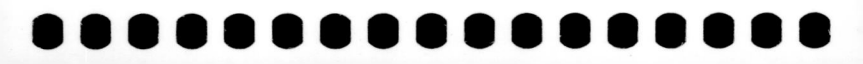

Leaves: © javarman/ShutterStock, Inc.

■ Marine-Animal Injuries

A treatment useful for one jellyfish species may worsen a sting from another jellyfish species. This contributes to confusion about what treatment is best for stings. Check with local experts, if possible.

For example, confusion exists about using vinegar to treat jellyfish stings. A review of 19 reputable medical articles (*Annals of Emergency Medicine* 2012;60:399–414), says vinegar increases pain or nematocyst discharge in most jellyfish species and therefore should not be used.

Injury Type	Marine Animal	What to Do
Bite, rip, or puncture	Sharks Barracudas Eels	1. Control bleeding. 2. Wash the wound with soap and water. 3. Flush the area with water under pressure. 4. Treat for shock. 5. Seek medical help. *(continued)*

| Sting | Jellyfish
Portuguese man-of-wars
Sea anemone
Fire coral | For North American oceans:
1. **Immediately remove tentacles.** Tentacles may detach and stick to the skin. Remove them as soon as possible by washing the affected skin with seawater for at least 30 seconds. Avoid using fresh water because it may activate the venomous stingers (nematocysts) that are embedded in the skin.
• **DO NOT** touch the tentacles with your hands.
• **DO NOT** try to rub the tentacles off with a towel or clothing because it may cause the discharge of more venom. Removing tentacles with tweezers may also discharge more venom. |

(continued)

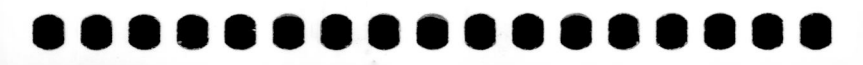

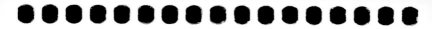

2. **DO NOT** attempt to deactivate stingers unless you know what type of jellyfish it is and how to deactivate it. Deactivation of stingers is controversial partly because how to deactivate depends on the species of jellyfish. What works for one may make another worse. Vinegar may be used on Portuguese man-of-war stings.

3. **Relieve pain or irritation.** Once all tentacles are removed by flushing with salt water, warm fresh water may help to deactivate the toxins. Use non-scalding hot water either by a shower or immersing for at least 20 minutes for all jellyfish stings in North America and Hawaii. Xylocaine (Lidocaine), an over-the-counter medication, can be applied on the affected skin.

(continued)

		DO NOT use the following remedies because research does not support them or they have been shown to be ineffective: human urine, meat tenderizer, alcohol, and pressure bandages.
Sting	Sea snake Octopus Cone shell	1. Apply a compression bandage on the entire bitten arm or leg. 2. Seek medical help.
Puncture (by spine)	Stingray Scorpion fish Stonefish Starfish Catfish	1. Relieve pain by immersing affected part in hot water for 30 to 90 minutes or until pain subsides. **DO NOT** use water hot enough to cause a burn. 2. Wash the wound with soap and water. 3. Flush the area with water under pressure. 4. Treat the wound.

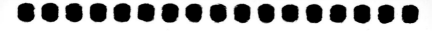

■ Motion Sickness

What to Look for

Occurs while traveling by car, truck, van, bus, train, ship, or airplane
- Sweating
- Dizziness
- Pale skin
- Nausea, sometimes leading to vomiting

What to Do

1. Stop activity if possible.
2. Give over-the-counter antinausea pills (such as Dramamine or Bonine).
3. Give ginger, either as a solid or liquid, or in capsules taken on an empty stomach.
4. Use thumb pressure or an acupressure wristband (Sea-Band or Psi Band) to apply pressure in the center of the wrist between the two forearm bones, two finger widths from the wrist crease. Press three to five times firmly for 1 minute, and then repeat on the other arm.

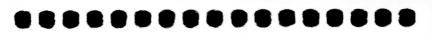

N

Leaves: © javarman/Shutterstock, Inc.

■ Nose Injuries

What to Look for	What to Do
Broken nose	1. If bleeding, care for the nosebleed. 2. Apply cold for 15 minutes. 3. Medical help can be delayed. 4. **DO NOT** try to straighten a crooked nose.
Nosebleed	1. If nose was hit, suspect a broken nose. 2. Have victim sit leaning slightly forward. 3. Pinch nostrils together for 10 minutes. 4. If bleeding has not stopped, have victim gently blow nose to get rid of ineffective blood clots. Pinch nostrils together again for 10 minutes. 5. Try other methods in addition to nose pinching, such as applying an ice pack or spraying decongestant spray in nostrils. 6. Medical help is not usually needed. If bleeding continues, seek medical help.

(continued)

What to Look for	What to Do
Foreign object (a problem mainly with children)	Try one or more of these methods to remove an object: • Have victim gently blow nose while compressing the opposite nostril. • If an object is visible, pull the object out with tweezers. **DO NOT** push object deeper. • Induce sneezing by sniffing pepper. • Seek medical help if the object cannot be removed.

Leaves: © javarman/ShutterStock, Inc.

Plant-Related Problems

Plant-Induced Dermatitis: Poison Ivy, Poison Oak, and Poison Sumac

Poison ivy can be found in every state, except Hawaii and Alaska. Poison oak grows in some eastern states and along the West Coast. Poison sumac is found mainly in swampy areas on the East Coast, especially in the Southeast.

Poison ivy growing in one area may not look anything like poison ivy found halfway across the country, and poison oak of the East is very different from poison oak in the West. However, the dermatitis that these plants cause—and the treatment—is similar. **Figure 20**

About 50% of the people exposed to these plants break out in a rash. The "poison" in these plants is the chemical urushiol, which is found in the sap. All parts of the plant— leaves, stems, roots, flowers, and berries—contain urushiol oil.

An allergic reaction may begin as early as 6 hours after exposure with a line of small blisters where the skin brushed

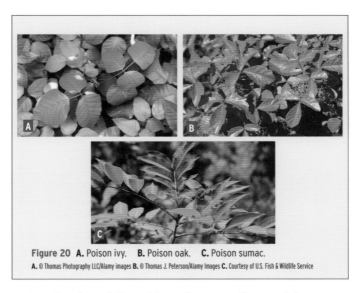

Figure 20 A. Poison ivy. **B.** Poison oak. **C.** Poison sumac.

A. © Thomas Photography LLC/Alamy images **B.** © Thomas J. Peterson/Alamy Images **C.** Courtesy of U.S. Fish & Wildlife Service

against the plant, followed by redness, swelling, and larger blisters. The blister fluid does not contain the irritant. Usually, the onset of symptoms is 24 to 72 hours after exposure.

As long as 2 weeks after the initial eruption, the rash may appear on other areas of the body. This can be explained by either (1) skin that was exposed to less urushiol or (2) that different parts of the body absorb and react differently to urushiol.

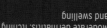

Poison ivy, oak, and sumac dermatitis are self-limiting conditions. Without any treatment, a mild case of any of these will often disappear in about 2 weeks. Usually the discomfort is significant, and the first aid procedures discussed here do not cure the condition but simply ease the suffering. Over-the-counter hydrocortisone cream or ointment (1%) offers little benefit. Seek medical advice for severe cases. Do not worry about spreading the rash to others; it is not contagious. However, animals can carry the oil on their fur and smoke from burning plants can carry particles of the oil. Both can affect an allergic person.

What to Look for	What to Do
Known contact within 5 minutes for people with sensitive skin and up to 1 hour for people with moderately sensitive skin	Wash skin with soap and lots of water or rubbing alcohol (isopropyl). **DO NOT** dab it on or use pre-packaged alcohol wipes.
Mild dermatitis: itching	Use any of the following methods • Oatmeal soaks (Aveeno Soothing Bath Treatments) • Calamine lotion • Burow's solution (Domeboro [aluminum acetate]) • Baking soda paste (1 teaspoon of water mixed with 3 teaspoons of baking soda)
Moderate dermatitis: itching and swelling	• Same as for mild signs and symptoms • Physician-prescribed cortisone ointment (continued)

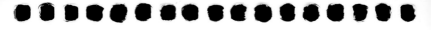

What to Look for	What to Do
Severe dermatitis: itching, swelling, and blisters	• Same as for mild and moderate symptoms • Physician-prescribed topical or oral cortisone • Seek medical help if smoke from a burning plant is inhaled or if the reaction involves the face, eyes, genitals, or large areas of the body.

Cactus Spines

Cacti grow in hot, sunny, dry environments. They grow in many sizes and shapes and are usually covered in spines or needles. When the skin is pricked, it causes pain and redness. If not removed, the skin can become inflamed and infected.

What to Look for	What to Do
Medium or large spine(s) embedded in the skin	Remove with tweezers or pliers by: 1. Grasping the spine close to the skin. 2. Slowly pulling the spine out in the same direction that the spine entered. Clean and treat the small wound with antibiotic ointment and dressing. *(continued)*

What to Look for

Hair-like small needles (numbering in the dozens to hundreds) embedded in the skin

What to Do

When combined, steps 1 and 2 below are considered to be the most effective method for removing most of the needles.
1. Remove as many needles as you can with tweezers. A magnifying glass may help locate the needles. This method will not remove all small needles.
2. Use glue. Spread a thin layer of white wood-working glue (i.e., Elmer's Glue-All) or rubber cement onto the affected area. **DO NOT** use Super Glue. Press gauze over the glue and wait for it to dry (30 minutes). Gently roll or pull the gauze up from the skin.
3. Try using duct tape (may remove up to 30% of the needles even after many attempts). Stretch a piece of duct tape over the affected area. Press the duct tape onto the skin and gently rub it over the needles to make sure they are stuck. Grasp one end of the tape and quickly rip it off. Repeat with fresh pieces of tape. Adhesive tape and cellophane tape are not very effective.

(continued)

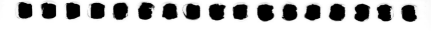

What to Look for	What to Do
	4. If a cactus stem or pad is attached, use a plastic comb or two sticks to grasp underneath the stem or pad and flick it away before trying any of the above methods. **DO NOT** allow the victim to suck needles out because they can lodge in the tongue, gums, or throat. 5. Clean and treat the wound with antibiotic ointment and dressing.

Stinging Nettle

The stinging nettle plant has stinging hairs on its stem and leaves. Its effects are not an allergic response but are due to an irritant found in the plant's sap.

What to Look for	What to Do
Immediate onset of intense burning sensation; itching	1. Wash the area with soap and water. 2. Apply a cold, wet pack. You could also use colloidal oatmeal, hydrocortisone cream (1%), or calamine lotion. 3. Give an antihistamine, if desired, following the package directions.

Swallowed (Ingested) Poisonous Plant

What to Look for

- Abdominal pain and cramping
- Nausea or vomiting
- Diarrhea
- Drowsiness

What to Do

1. Rapidly determine:
   - The type of plant, if possible
   - How much was swallowed
   - When it was swallowed
2. For an alert, responsive victim, use a cell phone if available and call the national poison control center (the national number is 1-800-222-1222). Most poisonings can be treated through telephone instructions.
3. For an unresponsive victim, check breathing and treat accordingly. Seek medical help ASAP.
4. Place the victim on his/her left side to delay poison's advance into the small intestine.
5. **DO NOT** try to induce vomiting.
6. Seek medical help ASAP for all mushroom-poisoned victims.

S

Seizures

Seizures result from a disturbance of the electrical activity in the brain, causing uncontrollable muscle movements. Causes include epilepsy, head injury, brain tumor, stroke, heatstroke, poisoning (including alcohol or drugs), insulin reaction, or high fever.

What to Look for	What to Do

• A sudden cry or scream
• A sudden loss of responsiveness
• Rigid body followed by jerky movement with arching of the back (convulsions)
• Foaming at mouth
• Drooling from mouth
• Grinding of teeth
• Face and lips turn blue
• Eyes roll upward
• Loss of bladder or bowel control
	1. Protect the victim from injury. Place something flat and soft under the head.
	2. Loosen restrictive, tight clothing.
	3. **DO NOT** open or place anything into the victim's mouth.
	4. **DO NOT** restrain the victim.
	5. Roll victim onto side to drain fluids.
	6. Seek medical help if any of these apply:
	  • Nonepileptic victim
	  • A seizure lasting more than 5 minutes
	  • First-time seizure
	  • Slow recovery
	  • Pregnant victim
	
	(continued)

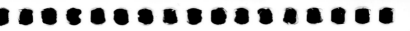

■ Shock

Shock happens when the body's tissues do not get enough blood. Do not confuse this with an electric shock or "being shocked," as in scared or surprised. Shock is life threatening. Even if there are no signs of shock, you should still follow these procedures for injured victims.

What to Look for	What to Do
Altered mental status: anxiety and restlessness • Pale, cold, and clammy skin, lips, and nail beds • Nausea/vomiting • Rapid breathing and heart rate • Unresponsiveness when shock is severe	1. Treat injuries. 2. If responsive, lay the victim down. If unresponsive, roll the victim on his/her side. If a spinal injury is suspected, while rolling the victim, keep his/her nose and navel pointing in the same direction. 3. Prevent body heat loss by putting blankets/coats under and over victim. 4. If the victim does not improve, seek medical help. **DO NOT** give anything to eat or drink unless medical help is delayed over 1 hour, in which case, sips of water can be given if fluids do not cause nausea and/or vomiting.

What to Look for	What to Do
• Injury related • Multiple seizures in a row with incomplete recovery in between	

Snake and Other Reptile Bites

In about 25% of venomous snakebites, there is no venom injected, only fang and tooth wounds (known as a "dry" bite).
For all snake and reptile bites:

- Get the victim and bystanders away from the snake or reptile because of the risk of a second bite. A dead snake can still bite even if decapitated.
- Keep the victim quiet and still.
- Gently wash the bite with soap and water.

Reptile	What to Look for	What to Do
Pit Vipers **Figure 21** · Rattlesnakes · Copperheads · Cottonmouths/ Water Moccasins Triangular, flat head, wider than the neck; vertical, elliptical pupils (cat's eye); and a heat-sensitive "pit" located between the eye and nostril	· Severe, burning pain at the bite site · Two small puncture wounds (victim may have only one) · Swelling within 10 to 15 minutes; can involve entire extremity · Discoloration and blood-filled blisters possible in 6 to 10 hours · Severe cases have nausea, vomiting, sweating, and weakness	1. It is not necessary to identify or kill the snake. 2. Seek medical help. When possible, carry the victim. If alone and capable, walk slowly. *Cautions:* **DO NOT** cut the victim's skin to drain venom. **DO NOT** use mouth suction. **DO NOT** use any suction device. **DO NOT** apply cold/ice packs. **DO NOT** give alcohol.

(continued)

Reptile	What to Look for	What to Do
		DO NOT apply electrical shock. **DO NOT** use a tourniquet.

Coral snakes Small and very colorful, with a series of bright red, yellow, and black bands going all the way around its body. Every alternate band is yellow, and the snout is black. It is the most venomous snake in North America, but rarely bites.	• Few immediate signs
	• Absence of immediate symptoms is not evidence of a harmless bite.
	• Several hours may pass before the onset of:
	  • Nausea
	  • Vomiting
	  • Sweating
	  • Tremors
	  • Drowsiness
	  • Slurred speech
	  • Blurred vision
	  • Swallowing difficulty
	  • Breathing difficulty
		1. Apply mild pressure by wrapping several elastic bandages (e.g., Ace) over the bite site and entire extremity.
		2. **DO NOT** cut skin or use suction.
		3. Seek medical help.

Nonvenomous snakes Figure 22 If in doubt, assume that the snake is venomous.	• Leaves a horseshoe shape of tooth marks on skin • Possible swelling and tenderness	1. Treat the bite the same as a shallow wound. (Refer to *Bleeding and Wound Care* section). 2. Consult with a physician.
Venomous lizards • Gila monster (U.S. and Mexico) • Mexican bearded lizard	• Puncture wounds–teeth may break off • Swelling and pain, often severe and burning • Sweating	1. Give pain medication. 2. Seek medical help. 3. Same as Pit Vipers.

Reptile	What to Look for	What to Do
May firmly hang on during bite and chew venom into skin	• Vomiting • Increased heart rate • Shortness of breath	

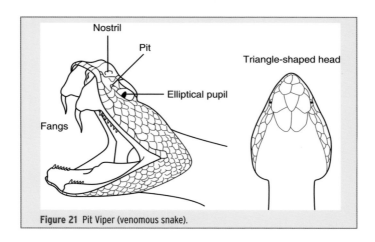

Figure 21 Pit Viper (venomous snake).

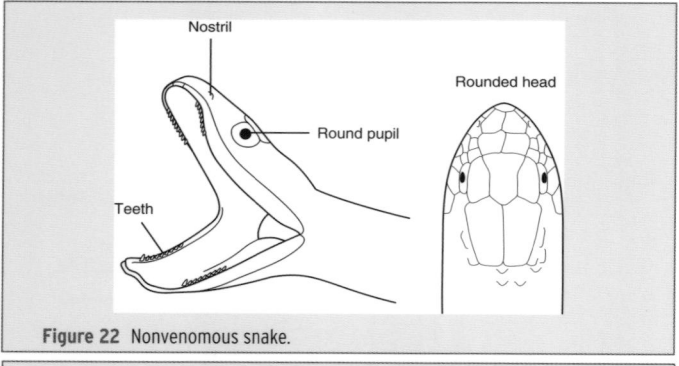

Figure 22 Nonvenomous snake.

Nostril

Round pupil

Rounded head

Teeth

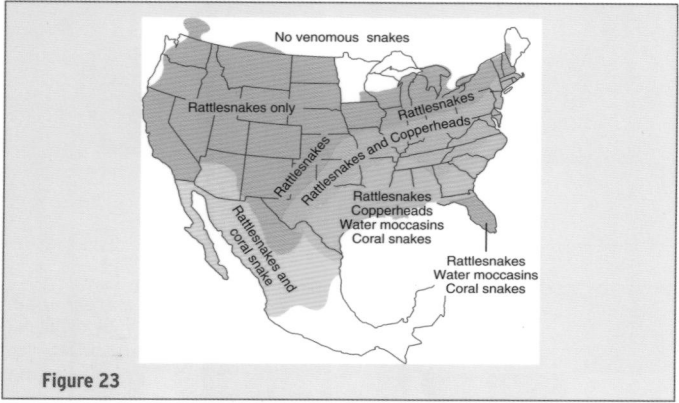

No venomous snakes

Rattlesnakes only

Rattlesnakes

Rattlesnakes and Copperheads

Rattlesnakes
Copperheads
Water moccasins
Coral snakes

Rattlesnakes and coral snake

Rattlesnakes
Water moccasins
Coral snakes

Figure 23

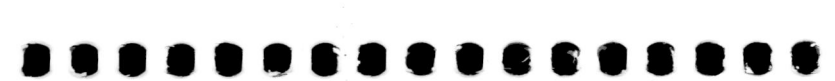

■ Spinal Injury

When a significant cause of injury (e.g., a vehicle crash involving ejection, a rollover, or high speeds; a head injury causing unresponsiveness; penetrating wounds of the neck or trunk; or diving into shallow water) occurs, always suspect a spinal injury.

Fully stabilizing a responsive person may not always be necessary, because doing so can be difficult, impractical, impossible, or dangerous to the victim.

A *reliable* victim does not need to be stabilized in one position if he or she meets the following criteria:

- Alert, knows name and where he or she is
- Not intoxicated by drugs/alcohol
- Calm, cooperative
- Lack of painful, distracting injury

An *unreliable* victim meets one or more of the following criteria:

- Unresponsive; altered mental status
- Intoxicated by drugs/alcohol
- Combative, confused
- Has a painful, distracting injury

What to Look for

In a reliable victim:
1. Reports back pain and leg numbness and tingling
2. Tenderness/pain when you run fingers all the way down spine (if possible); press each bump of vertebrae and press on depressions produced on each side when you touch or push on the spine bones.

3. Fails these tests for sensation and movement (test all four extremities):
   - Upper body:
     a. Pinch several fingers and ask: "Can you feel this? Where am I touching you?"
     b. Ask: "Can you wiggle your fingers?"
     c. Have victim squeeze your hand.
   - Lower body:
     a. Pinch toes and ask: "Can you feel this? Where am I touching you?"
     b. Ask: "Can you wiggle your toes?"

What to Do

Suspect a spinal injury:
1. Send for medical help. **DO NOT** attempt to evacuate the victim. Wait for trained rescuers with proper equipment.
2. Leave the victim on the ground. Cover to prevent heat loss by log rolling the victim, keeping nose and navel pointing in the same direction, and place insulating materials under and over the victim.

3. Stabilize victim against movement. Place the victim's head between your knees, as this is less tiring than kneeling and holding the victim's head with your hands. Improvised cervical collars (e.g., SAM Splint, blanket) alone are inadequate. An alternative method that does not require you to hold the victim constantly is to improvise "sandbags" by placing dirt, sand, or rocks cushioned with clothing in stuff sacks or plastic bags and securely placing them on both sides of the victim's head.

(continued)

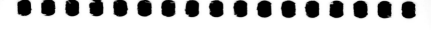

What to Look for	What to Do
c. Have the victim push and pull a foot against your hand.	
If these are *not* present in a reliable victim	Suspect *no* spinal injury. Treat other injuries (e.g., wounds, bruises, fractures).
If the victim is unreliable and has a significant mechanism of injury (see above for examples)	Assume that there is a spinal injury. Use the methods given above to stabilize the victim.

An injured victim does not require spinal stabilization if he or she:

- Is alert, not intoxicated, and has no distracting injuries
- Does not report neck pain or neurological symptoms (e.g., tingling, numbness)
- Has no neck tenderness when felt, no loss of sensation when fingers and toes are pinched, and can move the fingers and toes
- Can rotate neck 45 degrees left and right when requested.

■ Stroke ("Brain Attack")

Stroke is caused by blockage or rupture of a blood vessel in the brain.

A stroke occurs when a brain blood vessel becomes plugged or ruptures so that part of the brain does not get the blood flow it needs.

What to Look for

The acronym **FAST** provides an assessment to determine if a stroke may have occurred:

F – **Face**: Ask the victim to smile. It is abnormal to have one side of face not move well compared with the other side.

A – **Arm drift**: Ask the victim to raise both arms. It is abnormal if one arm drifts downward when held extended.

S – **Speech**: Ask the victim to repeat a simple phrase (i.e., "The sky is blue."). It is abnormal if the victim slurs words, uses the wrong word, or cannot speak at all.

T – **Time** to seek medical help if any of the above signs occur. Presence of one of the above is associated with a high risk of stroke (72%); if all three are present, the risk is 85%.

What to Do

1. Monitor breathing. If victim not breathing, begin CPR.
2. Position the victim on his/her back with head and shoulders slightly raised.
3. Loosen tight or constricting clothing.
4. Be prepared to turn the victim onto his/her side to allow drool or vomit to drain.
5. If unresponsive but breathing, place victim on his/her side.
6. Seek medical help ASAP.

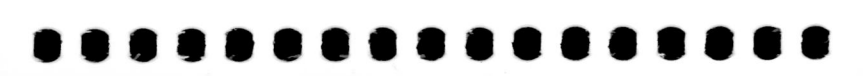

Leaves: © javarman/ShutterStock, Inc.

Tooth Injuries

What to Look for	What to Do
Toothache	1. Rinse victim's mouth with warm water.
	2. Remove trapped food with dental floss.
	3. Use a cold pack on the outside of the cheek to reduce swelling.
	4. If available, use a cotton swab to paint the aching tooth with oil of cloves (eugenol).
	5. **DO NOT** place aspirin on aching tooth or gum tissue.
	6. Give pain medication (e.g., aspirin, acetaminophen, or ibuprofen).
	7. Seek a dentist.
Broken tooth	1. Rinse victim's mouth with warm water.
	2. Apply cold pack to the outside of the face to decrease swelling.
	3. If a jaw fracture is suspected, stabilize the jaw by wrapping a bandage under the chin and over the top of the head.
	4. Seek a dentist ASAP.
	(continued)

What to Look for	What to Do

What to Look for

Knocked-out tooth

What to Do

1. Find the tooth and handle it by the crown. O NOT touch the root.
2. If the tooth is dirty, rinse it with water. DO NOT scrub or remove any of the root's attached tissue fragments.
3. Replace tooth into its socket. A tooth can usually be saved if cared for properly and reimplanted within 1 hour. Make sure it faces the right way and never force it into the socket. Push down on the tooth so the top is even with adjacent teeth. Have the victim bite down gently on gauze or handkerchief placed between the teeth.
4. If step 3 above is not possible, use one of the following methods for storing a tooth until a dentist is available:
   a) Place tooth in a tooth preservation product that has the American Dental Association Seal of Acceptance (i.e., Save-a-Tooth), or
   b) Transport tooth in the victim's mouth, keeping it between the molars and the inside of the cheek, or
   c) Have the victim spit in a small container and place the tooth in it, or
   d) Place the tooth in a small container of cold whole milk.
   DO NOT store the tooth in water.
5. Seek a dentist ASAP.

(continued)

What to Look for	What to Do
Infected or abscessed tooth · Swelling of the gums around the affected tooth · Foul breath · Pain that is increased by tapping the tooth with something metal (i.e., spoon handle)	1. Have victim rinse his/her mouth several times a day with warm water. 2. Give pain medication. **DO NOT** suck or place an aspirin on the tooth or gum tissue. 3. A cold pack on the cheek may help. 4. Remove trapped food with dental floss. 5. Seek a dentist.
Cavity-caused by decay or lost filling · Sensitivity to heat, cold, or sweets · Sensitivity to touch. Tap the tooth gently with something metal (i.e., spoon handle) on the top and side. This increases the pain in the affected tooth.	1. Have victim rinse his/her mouth with warm water. 2. Apply oil of cloves (eugenol) with a cotton swab to the cavity to deaden the pain. **DO NOT** apply any on the gums, lips, or inside the cheeks. 3. If available, apply a temporary filling with cavity dental filling paste. Other options include sugarless chewing gum, candle wax, or ski wax. 4. Seek a dentist.

W

■ Wild Animal Attacks

Human injuries by wild animals are rare, yet people often have fear and apprehension about venturing into wild areas. Many of these reactions come from myths, ignorance, exaggeration, and sensationalism. Most wild animals try to avoid people, and when attacks do occur, they often result in only minor injuries. Traveling in a group is safer than being alone. In North America, the wild animals that are most commonly reported as interacting with people include bears, bison, moose, cougars, coyotes, and alligators. Not all injuries are bites. Severe injuries can result from victims being thrown in the air, gored by antlers, butted, or trampled on the ground. Injuries include puncture wounds, bites, lacerations, bruises, fractures, rupture of internal organs, and evisceration. The majority of wild animal attacks occur outside of the United States (for "What to Do," see the *Bleeding and Wound Care* section). Seek medical help ASAP.

Prevention

■ Prevention: Altitude Illness

1. **DO NOT** rush to your destination. At higher elevations, start slowly and avoid overexertion. Those not accustomed to high altitudes should not ascend rapidly to sleeping altitudes greater than 10,000 feet and should spend 2 to 3 nights at 8,000 to 10,000 feet before going higher, with 1 extra night for every 2,000 to 3,000 feet. You can climb or ski higher during the day and return to a lower elevation at night ("climb or ski high, sleep low").
2. Drink lots of water (see the *Prevention: Dehydration* section for information).
3. Eat a high-carbohydrate diet because the appetite is often suppressed; also, food may be less available, and energy needs are greater.
4. **DO NOT** take sleeping pills because they cause shallow breathing while sleeping.
5. **DO NOT** smoke because it increases carbon monoxide blood levels, lessening the body's ability to use oxygen.

6. Ask your physician about the possible use of the medication acetazolamide (Diamox), which can prevent symptoms of acute mountain illness.

■ Prevention: Avalanche Burial

An avalanche is a mass of snow that slides down a mountainside.

1. Before going into potential avalanche country, call the nearest avalanche hotline to get the latest information about mountain weather, snow, and avalanche conditions.

2. Only one person at a time should go onto a slope that looks risky. Other people should serve as spotters from a safe location.

3. Avoid the center of open slopes. Cross an open slope at the very top or bottom.

4. Stay on shallow slopes. Avalanches most often start on slopes that are 30 to 45 degrees. Areas where avalanches occur year after year should be avoided. **Figure 24**

5. **DO NOT** travel alone.

6. If caught in an avalanche:

- Try to escape to the side of the avalanche. **DO NOT** try to outrun by going downhill on skis or snowmobile.
- Try to grab a tree.

- Try to swim with the moving snow, similar to body surfing in the ocean.
- Try to get away from a snowmobile, and get rid of ski poles.
- Try to burst through the surface before the avalanche stops and clear a breathing space over your mouth.

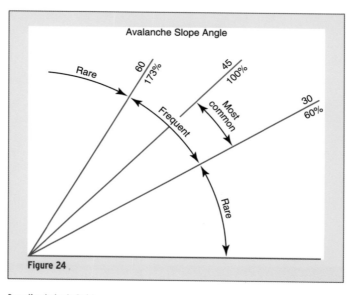

Figure 24

■ Prevention: Bear Attack

Bear attacks rarely happen. Most encounters end without injury.

1. Avoid areas where high bear activity has been recently reported.
2. Try to avoid surprising a bear by making noise; hike with a group.
3. Hike during daylight hours.
4. Recognize the signs of a bear (e.g., footprints, droppings, and scratches against trees with hair left).
5. Avoid using highly odorous foods that may attract a bear.
6. Properly store your food and garbage at all times except when they are being transported, prepared, or used. Store all food in vehicles or high in a tree—away from the sleeping area. Deposit garbage in a refuse container or store as you would food. **DO NOT** bury it.
7. Never feed bears; never approach bears.
8. If a bear charges you:
   - **DO NOT** run—you cannot outrun a bear; try to remain calm.
   - **DO NOT** climb a tree—black bears and young grizzlies can climb trees.
   - **DO NOT** make quick movements; talk to the bear in a normal, monotone voice.
   - **DO NOT** stare directly at the bear.

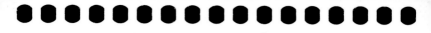

- If you have pepper spray, prepare to use it.
- If the bear makes a bluff charge, stand quietly in a nonaggressive stance. In most cases, the bear stops the charge without making contact or causing injury. At this point, leave the area in the opposite direction from the bear.
- For a black bear without cubs, try to chase it off with mild aggression—yell, shout, blow a whistle, throw rocks, and bang pots. If the bear does not leave, back away and leave the area.

9. During an attack:
   - Keep a backpack on for protection.
   - If you have pepper spray (oil-based capsaicin), spray the bear's eyes when the bear gets within about 20 feet. Continue spraying until the bear stops its charge; the spray lasts from four to nine seconds.
   - If it is a black bear, fight back by yelling, throwing rocks or sticks or whatever is available, and hitting and gouging the bear with your feet, fists, sticks, rocks, shovels—anything you have. **Figure 25**
   - If it is a brown bear (grizzly, Kodiak), play dead. Drop to the ground as the bear touches you—not before— and curl into a ball, covering your neck and head with your hands and arms. **DO NOT** struggle or fight back, and keep quiet. If the bear swats at you, roll with it.

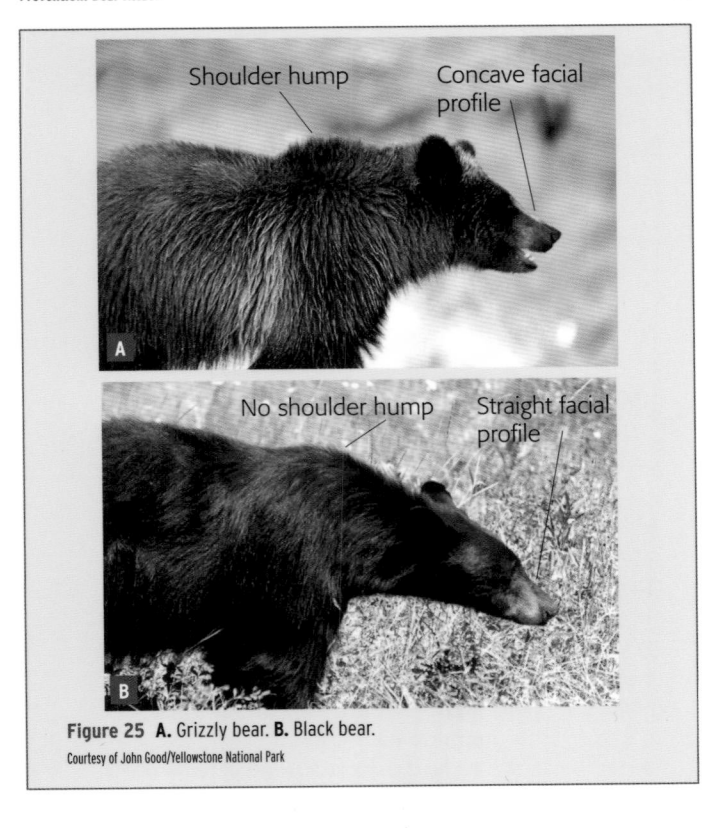

Figure 25 A. Grizzly bear. **B.** Black bear.
Courtesy of John Good/Yellowstone National Park

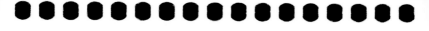

Stay facedown and **DO NOT** look around, and **DO NOT** get up until you are sure it is gone.

If any bear preys on you, try to get away, shout for help, fight for your life, and defend yourself with anything available.

■ Prevention: Blisters

1. Buy shoes or boots with adequate room in the toe box and with a good fit in the heel. They should be a size to a size and half larger than your dress shoes.
2. Wear socks made of a moisture-wicking fabric (CoolMax) or polypropylene next to the foot to wick moisture away from the foot. Corn starch, talcum powder, baby powder, and antiperspirant also help to keep feet dry.
3. Wear a second pair of socks to prevent friction on the foot itself. Do not wear cotton socks.
4. Coat areas of the feet prone to blister with a blister–chafing prevention agent such as petroleum jelly or A & D (per company website) ointment.
5. For areas that are already raw or very prone to blister, cover with moleskin.
6. Stop whenever you feel a hot spot developing, and cover the area with moleskin, molefoam, athletic tape, or duct tape.
7. Change wet socks into dry ones when possible.

■ Prevention: Cold-Related Emergencies (Adapted from the Colorado Mountain Club)

If venturing into the wilderness in cold weather, you should have, at a minimum, a wire saw, fire starter, and a Mylar emergency blanket.

Seek and create shelter from cold, wind, snow, and rain:

1. If possible, retreat to timbered areas for shelter construction and fire.
2. Use natural shelters: the windless side of ridges, rock croppings, slope depressions, snow blocks, a snow hole at the base of standing trees, dense stands of trees, or downed trees.
3. Improvise a windbreak or shelter from stacked rocks or snow blocks, tree trunks, limbs, and bark slabs and evergreen boughs, or dig a snow cave or snow trench with a cover. **Figure 26**

Conserve, Share, and Create Warmth

1. Conserve body heat by putting on extra clothing. Replace damp clothing and socks. Loosen boot laces to increase circulation. Use a sleeping pad (Ensolite) or evergreen boughs to insulate the body from the ground. Place hands in your armpits or crotch.

Windchill Chart

Temperature (°F)																		
Calm	40	35	30	25	20	15	10	5	0	−5	−10	−15	−20	−25	−30	−35	−40	−45
5	36	31	25	19	13	7	1	−5	−11	−16	−22	−28	−34	−40	−46	−52	−57	−63
10	34	27	21	15	9	−4	−4	−10	−16	−22	−28	−35	−41	−47	−53	−59	−66	−72
15	32	25	19	13	6	−7	−7	−13	−19	−26	−32	−39	−45	−51	−58	−64	−71	−77
20	30	24	17	11	4	−9	−9	−15	−22	−29	−35	−42	−48	−55	−61	−68	−74	−81
25	29	23	16	9	3	−11	−11	−17	−24	−31	−37	−44	−51	−58	−64	−71	−78	−84
30	28	22	15	8	1	−12	−12	−19	−26	−33	−39	−46	−53	−60	−67	−73	−80	−87
35	28	21	14	7	0	−14	−14	−21	−27	−34	−41	−48	−55	−62	−69	−76	−82	−89
40	27	20	13	6	−1	−8	−15	−22	−29	−36	−43	−50	−57	−64	−71	−78	−84	−91
45	26	19	12	5	−2	−9	−16	−23	−30	−37	−44	−51	−58	−65	−72	−79	−86	−93
50	26	19	12	4	−3	−10	−17	−24	−31	−38	−45	−52	−60	−67	−74	−81	−88	−95
55	25	18	11	4	−3	−11	−18	−25	−32	−39	−46	−54	−61	−68	−75	−82	−89	−97
60	25	17	10	3	−4	−11	−19	−26	−33	−33	−33	−33	−33	−33	−76	−84	−91	−98

Wind (mph)

Frostbite Times ▢ 30 minutes ▢ 10 minutes ▢ 5 minutes

$$\text{Wind Chill (°F)} = 35.74 + 0.6215T - 35.75(V^{0.16}) + 0.4275T(V^{0.16})$$

Where, T=Air Temperature (°F) V=Wind Speed (mph)

Figure 26
Courtesy of NWS/NOAA

2. Share body heat. Sit or lie front to back or back to back. Warm the hands and feet of the injured person or companion.

3. Create body heat. Nibble high-energy goods—candy, nuts, or granola bar. Sip water that is kept warm with body heat. Use a solid fuel hand warmer, igniting both ends of fuel stick (good for 4 hours of heat). Do isometric exercises (exercises done in one position, such as hand

press; sit up with back straight and arms straight out in front, then grasp hands together and press firmly) to stir the body's circulation system.

4. Build a fire. Find dry wood—dead lower branches and bark from underside of trees. Look under downed trees and inside of dead logs for dry kindling. Wet wood will burn as it dries in a strong fire. Select a sheltered area, protected from strong winds, as the site for an emergency campfire. Under snow conditions, build a fire base first, with 4-inch diameter or larger pieces of wood (use wire saw). Put fire starter on the base. Surround the fire starter with branches to hold kindling above the fire starter, and then place a hatch work of kindling and slightly larger wood on the branches. Light the fire starter, and blow lightly to help its flame ignite kindling. Add progressively larger wood to the flame area.

5. **DO NOT** drink alcoholic beverages because they:
   - Cause frequent urination, resulting in dehydration
   - Dilate the skin's blood vessels, allowing more heat loss

6. Prevent heat loss. Remember that the body loses heat by respiration, evaporation, conduction, radiation, and convection.
   - To prevent loss by respiration, cover the mouth and nose with loosely woven wool or fleece.
   - To reduce evaporation through excessive perspiration, wear layers of clothing that allow your skin to breathe.

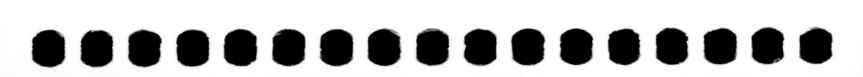

- To avoid loss by conduction, use a sleeping pad (Ensolite) and/or other cover between the body and a cold, wet surface. This insulation is particularly important if you are already wet.
- To prevent loss by radiation, keep the head, hands, and feet covered.
- To prevent loss by convection, protect the body from the wind. A Mylar emergency blanket is a very effective wind block and is also waterproof.

Clothing

1. Wear a base or first layer of clothing made of polypropylene.
2. Wear an insulating or second layer consisting of shirt and pants made of wool, fleece, or down.
3. Wear outer layers made of a windproof and water-resistant jacket that is worn loosely.
4. **DO NOT** wear cotton, as it does not wick sweat and will cool you rapidly if it gets wet.
5. Wear a stocking cap to insulate the head and retain heat. It should be large enough to cover the ears.
6. Wear a thin pair of gloves (or liners) inside a heavy wool or fleece mitten inside a Gore-Tex shell.
7. Remove layers as you warm up to prevent excessive sweating.

8.   Keep clothing dry from rain, snow, and sweat.

9.   **DO NOT** wear shoes or boots that are too small, or tie them so tightly that they restrict blood flow. **DO NOT** wear too many socks.

■ Prevention: Dehydration

The body operates more efficiently when it is well hydrated. Dehydration can increase the severity of most of the conditions described in this field guide, making them more difficult to deal with.

How Much Fluid to Drink?

The Institute of Medicine recommends 13 8-oz. cups of water and other beverages; for women, about 9 cups.

Pay special attention to fluid intake when:

- You are physically active.
- The air temperature exceeds 80°F.
- There is low humidity.
- You are at elevations above 5,000 feet.

How can you tell whether you are drinking enough?

- Check your urine—scanty, strong-smelling, dark urine signals that you need to drink more.
- Remember that the color of urine can be affected by medications, vitamins, and diet.

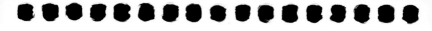

- If you feel thirsty, you are already about 1% to 2% dehydrated.

Can you drink too much water?

- If you overhydrate (drink too much), sodium concentrations can drop (hyponatremia), allowing water to leak into brain cells, causing headache, confusion, personality changes, and even seizures, coma, or death.
- During physical activity, stay within the range of about 1.5 to 3 cups per hour.

Can commercial sports drinks be used?

- During strenuous physical activity in hot environments lasting over 1 hour, commercial sport drinks may be used.
- **DO NOT** take salt tablets.
- Snack foods can be useful if they contain some sodium.

■ Prevention: Drowning (Submersion/Immersion)

1. Acquire swimming, rescue, and lifesaving skills.
2. Learn how to row a boat and paddle a raft and canoe safely.
3. Children should be supervised by an adult when they are near or in the water.
4. Everyone on a boat, canoe, or raft should wear a U.S. Coast Guard-approved life jacket that will support the person with the head above water, even if the person is unresponsive.

■ **Prevention: Heat Stress**

1. Keep as cool as possible.
   - Avoid direct sunlight when possible.
   - Wipe cool water on exposed areas of the skin and/ or place wet towels or ice bags on the body and/or dampen clothing.
   - Take cool baths or showers.
   - Dip clothing into water periodically, if possible.
2. Wear lightweight, porous, loose-fitting clothing that reflects heat, facilitates evaporative heat loss, and allows air to circulate around your body.
3. Wear a broad-brimmed hat.
4. Apply sunscreen with minimum SPF 15.
5. Avoid, when possible, strenuous physical activity, particularly in the sun and during the hottest part of the day.
6. Drink enough water. Drink 1 cup (8 oz.) every half hour during strenuous activity. (See *Prevention: Dehydration* section.)
7. **DO NOT** use salt tablets.
8. **DO NOT** drink alcoholic beverages (e.g., beer and wine).
9. Rest frequently in shade.
10. Adapt to the heat (acclimate) by exercising in the heat 60 to 90 minutes each day for 1 to 2 weeks.

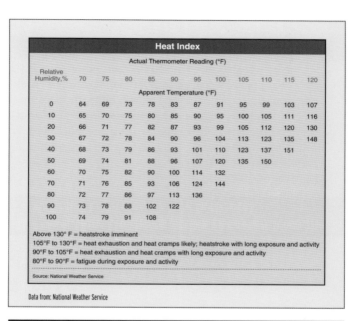

Heat Index

Actual Thermometer Reading (°F)

Relative Humidity,%	70	75	80	85	90	95	100	105	110	115	120
				Apparent Temperature (°F)							
0	64	69	73	78	83	87	91	95	99	103	107
10	65	70	75	80	85	90	95	100	105	111	116
20	66	71	77	82	87	93	99	105	112	120	130
30	67	72	78	84	90	96	104	113	123	135	148
40	68	73	79	86	93	101	110	123	137	151	
50	69	74	81	88	96	107	120	135	150		
60	70	75	82	90	100	114	132				
70	71	76	85	93	106	124	144				
80	72	77	86	97	113	136					
90	73	78	88	102	122						
100	74	79	91	108							

Above 130° F = heatstroke imminent
105°F to 130°F = heat exhaustion and heat cramps likely; heatstroke with long exposure and activity
90°F to 105°F = heat exhaustion and heat cramps with long exposure and activity
80°F to 90°F = fatigue during exposure and activity

Source: National Weather Service

Data from: National Weather Service

Prevention: Insect Stings (Bees, Wasps, Hornets, and Yellow Jackets)

1. **DO NOT** walk barefoot.
2. Insect repellents do not work against stinging insects.

3. **DO NOT** swat or flail at a flying insect. If need be, gently brush it aside or patiently wait for it to leave.
4. **DO NOT** drink from open beverage cans. Attracted by the sweet beverage, stinging insects will crawl inside a can.
5. When eating outdoors, try to keep food covered at all times.
6. **DO NOT** wear sweet-smelling perfumes, hair sprays, colognes, or deodorants.
7. **DO NOT** wear bright colored clothing with flowery patterns, which attracts flying insects.
8. Wear long pants and long-sleeved shirts.

■ Prevention: Lightning Strike (Adapted from the National Lightning Safety Institute)

If you can see lightning and/or hear thunder, you are already in danger. Louder or more frequent thunder indicates that lightning activity is approaching, increasing the risk for lightning injury or death. Estimate the distance in miles you are from a lightning flash by counting in seconds the time from when the flash is seen until the time the thunder is heard, and divide that number by five.

Use the "30-30 rule"—when the time between seeing the flash (lightning) and hearing the bang (thunder) is less than 30 seconds (this is the first "30"), meaning the lightning is less than 6 miles away, you should be in or seek a safer location. Outdoor

activities should not be resumed until at least 30 minutes (second "30") after the last lighting is seen or thunder heard.

1. When outdoors during a lightning/thunder storm:
   - Avoid water (lakes, rivers, etc.).
   - Avoid high ground.
   - Avoid open spaces where you are one of the tallest objects.
   - Avoid a single tree or other high object (e.g., rock and bush).
   - Avoid all metal objects including fences, machinery, etc.
   - Avoid small, isolated sheds, rain shelters, etc.

When possible, find shelter in a substantial building or in a fully enclosed metal vehicle such as a car or truck with the windows completely shut. **DO NOT** touch any of the vehicle's interior metal.

2. If lightning is striking nearby when you are outside:
   - Squat like a baseball catcher. Put your feet together. Place your hands over ears to minimize hearing damage from thunder. **DO NOT** lie flat on the ground because the current from a lightning strike can spread widely.
   - A group of people should spread out and stay a minimum of 15 feet apart.

3. If caught outdoors and no shelter is nearby:
   - Find a low spot away from trees, fences, and poles.
   - If you are in a forest, take shelter under the shorter trees or low brush.

- If you feel your skin tingle or hair stand on end, squat down like a baseball catcher.
4. If boating, try to get to shore as soon as possible.
5. When indoors:
   - Stay away from fireplaces, metal pipes, and open doors and windows.
   - **DO NOT** use a plugged-in telephone (cell phones are safe).
   - Turn off, unplug, and stay away from appliances, power tools, TV sets, etc.

Prevention: Mosquito Bites

1. Wear protective clothing during dawn and dusk or in areas where mosquitoes are active: long pants, long-sleeved shirt, and socks and shoes. For some areas, consider mosquito netting draped over a hat to protect face and neck.
2. Apply insect repellent containing DEET on exposed skin. **DO NOT** use a product with more than 30% DEET. **DO NOT** exceed 10% DEET for children under 5 years of age.
3. Apply permethrin only on clothing, not on the skin (permethrin kills insects; it is not a repellant).
4. Limit outdoor activities or take precautions given above at dawn and dusk.

■ Prevention: Mountain Lion Attack

1. Travel with others.
2. Keep small children close.
3. Obey warning signs or notices of mountain lion activity.
4. If you encounter a mountain lion:
   - **DO NOT** approach it; slowly back away. **DO NOT** turn your back to it.
   - **DO NOT** run—it may trigger an attack.
   - **DO NOT** make direct eye contact.
   - Appear larger than you are—raise arms above your head and make steady waving motions.
   - Yell or shout.
   - If small children are with you, pick them up.
   - If attacked, use anything as a weapon—a rock, branch, knife, or other hard object. If you have it, use pepper spray (oil-based capsaicin).

■ Prevention: Poisonous Plant Dermatitis

1. Learn to recognize and avoid poison ivy, poison oak, and poison sumac.
2. Wear long pants and long-sleeve shirts as protective clothing.

3. Apply an appropriate over-the-counter barrier cream (e.g., Ivy Block, Work Shield). Replenish the barrier protection every 4 to 6 hours when possible.
4. Wash or dispose of all contaminated clothing.

■ Prevention: Snakebite

1. **DO NOT** handle venomous snakes—keep away but do not kill them.
2. **DO NOT** hike and camp in snake-infested areas; avoid caves, rock crevices, dens, stonewalls, and wood piles.
3. Watch where you sit and step; **DO NOT** sit on or step over logs until closely checked. **DO NOT** reach into holes or hidden ledges.
4. Wear protective gear such as boots, long pants, and long-sleeved shirts.
5. **DO NOT** handle a dead venomous snake. The reflex action of the jaws can still inflict a bite 20 minutes or more after the snake is dead, even if decapitated.
6. **DO NOT** surprise or corner a snake. Use a walking stick to prod uncleared ground, and make noise so that a snake can sense you coming.
7. Check bedding, clothing, and shoes/boots before use.

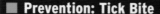

■ Prevention: Tick Bite

Ticks like to rest on low-lying brush and "catch a ride" on a passing animal or person. Areas with a high risk of ticks are wooded areas, low-growing grassland, and the seashore.

Ways to reduce chances of getting a tick bite include the following:

1. Avoid tick-infested areas, when possible.
2. In tick-infested areas, stay in the center of paths, avoid sitting on the ground, and check clothing.
3. Dress properly.
    -   Wear light-colored clothing so that ticks can be seen more easily and removed before becoming attached.
    -   Wear a long-sleeved shirt that fits tightly at the wrists and neck, and tuck your shirt into your pants.
    -   Wear long pants; tuck pant legs into boots or socks, or use masking or duct tape to secure pant legs tightly to socks, shoes, or boots.
4. After coming indoors, shower or bathe. Look and feel your entire body for ticks, especially in areas that have hair or where clothing was tight. Have a companion or use a mirror to check the scalp, behind and in the ears, neck, back, and behind the knees.

5. Use chemicals:
   - Apply insect repellents containing EPA-approved DEET to clothes and exposed skin. Avoid high-concentration products (more than 30% DEET) on the skin. **DO NOT** inhale or ingest DEET-containing products or get them in your eyes. **DO NOT** use products with more than 10% DEET on children under 5 years.
   - Apply 0.5% permethrin (kills ticks on contact) only to clothing and not the skin. Apply according to label instructions. Applications to shoes, socks, cuffs, and pant legs are most effective against ticks.

■ Prevention: Waterborne Diseases

There are three main ways of making water safe to drink: boiling, chemicals, and special filters. Before using any of these methods, cloudy or dirty water should first be filtered through a clean cloth or through an appropriate commercial filter.

Boiling

Bringing water to a full boil for 1 full minute at any altitude makes the water safe to drink.

Chemicals

Both iodine and chlorine are inexpensive and are available in tablet or liquid form. Iodine is preferred but should *not* be used if these conditions exist:

- Thyroid disease
- Iodine allergy
- Pregnancy

In all other people, it should not be used for more than a few months.

Iodine does not kill *Cryptosporidium*. Chemicals take longer to work in cold water and require larger amounts for cloudy or dirty water. Follow the manufacturer's directions concerning the amount administered.

Special Filters

Filters are expensive but simple to use. Filters are *not* a reliable method of removing viruses. (LifeStraw Personal Portable Water Filter is an example of a water filter that eliminates bacteria.)

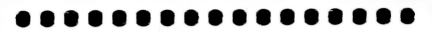

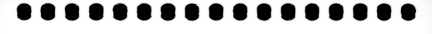

NOTES:

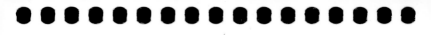

NOTES:

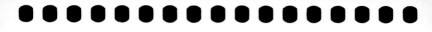

NOTES:

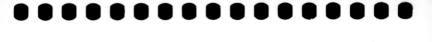